Dementia
A Positive Approach

Dementia
A Positive Approach

Lynne Phair
BSc(Hons), RGN, RMN, DPNS, MIFA

Valerie Good
BSc(Hons), CQSW, CertEd, DMS

With a foreword by
Professor Mary Marshall

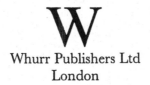

Whurr Publishers Ltd
London

© 1998 Whurr Publishers Ltd

First published 1995 by Scutari Press
Reprinted 1998 by Whurr Publishers Ltd
19b Compton Terrace, London N1 2UN, England

Reprinted 2001 and 2003

British Library Cataloguing in Publication data
A catalogue record for this book is available from the
British Library

ISBN 1 86156 081 8

Contents

Preface

Since qualifying we have both worked extensively in services providing care for older people with mental health problems. Over the years we have seen some improvements in this 'Cinderella' service and know of skilled and dedicated people trying to provide a quality service, often against a backdrop of prejudice, apathy and underfunding. We hope, by writing this book, both to encourage more people to work in this speciality and to give an impetus to those already in the field.

Recent developments have forced changes in the provision of continuing care beds in the NHS and long-stay beds in local authority 'Part III' homes. An ever-increasing number of older people with dementia are being cared for in the private and voluntary sectors and a growing number of joint services is developing, combining staff groups from both statutory agencies. Through writing this book we hope to show that the provision of high quality care for people with dementia is not the sole province of any one group. The fundamental requirements for quality care lie in appropriate attitudes and values. We can not provide sensitive care until we start to treat older people with dementia as we ourselves would wish to be treated.

We need to develop a service where staff can use a wide range of skills, anticipating difficulties before they become problems and dealing with them in a creative way. We want to encourage staff to reflect on their practice, try new ways of working and concentrate on caring for the person behind the illness.

Foreword

The writers of this useful book are fuelled by anger: anger at the discriminatory treatment many old people receive from supposedly caring services. This anger is quite appropriate. Indeed, without it you might be advised to work with another group of people. Working with older people, and even more so with people with dementia, is no bed of roses. Standards are tolerated which would be inconceivable with younger groups. Some of this discrimination is at the highest level.

It is seen, for example, in a willingness to spend the necessary money to house younger people with learning disabilities in houses for 3–4 residents; a number never considered 'economic' for people with dementia in spite of substantial evidence that smaller units have better outcomes in terms of functioning. Staff in this field have to be ready to go that extra mile in terms of pressing for better services while at the same time giving of their best to the people in their care.

Books like this one are important because they emphasise that working with people with dementia demands very high levels of skill. If we fail to provide these skills in the planning and management of care as well as in the front line, we condemn vulnerable people to a very poor quality of life.

We also deprive ourselves of rewarding work, because people with dementia are extraordinarily responsive in the positive (and negative) sense to the built and the social environment. We can really make a difference to their lives.

Those of us, like the authors of this book, who have worked for many years with older people remain excited and challenged by the opportunities it offers.

We enjoy learning all the time as new approaches and skills are developed. We relish the frustrations and the stimulation of working with colleagues from other professional groups. We derive great pleasure from the company of older people and in reflecting on our own old age. All of us experience ageing and most of us will experience old age. This alone should motivate us to ensure that the very best services and skills are available.

Professor Mary Marshall
Director, Dementia Services Development Unit
Stirling University, Scotland

Introduction

Dementia is a complex and fatal illness that causes devastating results in those it afflicts; in the last decade there have been exciting developments in our understanding of the disease process and researchers are moving closer to being able to pinpoint the causes of the illness. There have been parallel, but perhaps less well publicised, changes in our understanding of the kind of care that is most beneficial to people with dementia, with the development of some innovative practices, therapies and service delivery models.

In spite of this the care of older people is still considered by many to be an area of professional care where fewer skills are required; highly technical equipment is not needed and intricate laws, court cases and protection orders are not commonplace.

It is the belief of the authors that these attitudes have been supported by senior managers and policy makers within both health and social care settings. There are few areas in the health and social care field where such vulnerable people are cared for by the least qualified staff. For example, in the provision of residential care for children there have been recent moves to increase the number of staff holding professional qualifications, mainly in response to scandals over child abuse. Within health care, the Project 2000 curriculum does not include the speciality of caring for older people, while including the specialities of caring for children and adults.

There is a potent argument that says that it is ageist to have a separate service for older people and that everyone over the age of 18 is an adult. While respecting the argument, the reality is that any service so designed will focus on the needs of younger, more vocal people and that the needs of older people are likely to be overlooked. There are issues that are specific to older people and until we live in a society that has abandoned its ageist attitudes the care of older people will be best served by specialist units and specialist staff.

Good quality care is often measured in purely physical terms and quality assurance groups in most areas of inspection are still measuring physical phenomena, with little respect being paid to the older person and how they appear to be receiving the care, how the staff relate towards the older person and how care is structured to minimise incidents of aggression, 'wandering', incontinence or 'antisocial' behaviour. The reactive role of care professionals and their low self-esteem has seen the management of care become a problem-solving exercise rather than a proactive, creative process where planning and implementation are both rational and research based.

Imagine visiting two establishments offering care to older people with dementia. The first is a purpose-built building, newly opened with lavish furnishings. The second is a converted building that has been open for some time. Its furnishings and equipment are adequate and clean but not glamorous.

If you were attempting to decide which place offered the best care how much would the physical environment affect your decision? While it is important, most people would be equally interested in less visible attributes. These factors, the warmth and sensitivity of the staff, the 'atmosphere' and the ethos created and developed by the managers constitute the 'invisible quality' factor.

This book is aimed at helping you to improve your invisible quality factor while paying attention to improving the therapeutic value of the care environment. It also hopes to enable staff, whether in an institutional environment or working in a person's home, to be able to identify consciously methods of improving care and of minimising the risk of 'difficult to manage' behaviours arising.

Although it is important to be able to deal with problems it is far more effective and causes less distress to the older person if potential areas of difficulty can be identified and care designed, carers educated or staff attitudes developed that will diminish the chances of unwanted behaviour occurring.

The emphasis in this book is to look positively at the care of older people with a dementing illness and to examine the key aspects. Each subject area is discussed from a knowledge-based perspective and then readers are invited to reflect on their own practice and address the issues as they arise in their work environment.

Visitors to any service may appreciate the invisible quality factor but find it hard to define; the staff working in the service must be able to see the clear association of the invisible quality factor to a clearly articulated philosophy of care, a belief in a positive approach towards the care of older people and the demonstration of a high regard for staff working with older people.

You will find that each chapter begins with some key questions that will encourage you to start to think critically about your service and ends with an exploration of practical ways of bringing about change, with a constant emphasis on reflection and evaluation. The suggestions are only there to inspire and encourage; they are not meant to be exhaustive lists and not all the suggestions will be appropriate for you or the service in which you work.

The fundamental belief underlying the whole book is that many of the so-called 'problems' associated with dementia can be minimised or resolved through creative management.

Lynne Phair
Valerie Good

1 Attitudes

The relationship between beliefs and behaviour

Attitudes are important. There is a relationship between the attitudes of staff, the quality of the care they offer and the satisfaction that staff get from their job. It is important that social and professional attitudes to older people in general are identified as well as those specifically relating to older people who have dementia. Each professional group also has fixed and stereotypical beliefs about other professionals and good inter-agency working relies on an understanding of how these beliefs can help or hinder the establishment of effective relationships. The positive ways in which staff can show respect to the older person should be identified and the impact of an individual's feelings, fears and experiences of ageing and death should be examined.

POINTS TO PONDER

- How many of the staff in the unit are working with older people by choice?

- Compare the physical condition of your establishment to that of a unit for 'normal' old people. Is it as well equipped and furnished?

- How do the care professionals that work in your unit show that they value and respect older people with dementia?

- Think about an old person who regularly appears in a TV series? Do they portray a positive image of ageing?

- In your establishment do you spend more time considering how to minimise risks or safeguarding older people's rights?

- Can you think of a law that specifically protects the interests of older people?

- Can the staff group agree on 'how old is old'? Does anyone look forward to getting old? If so why?

- Can you remember what it felt to be 10 or 20 years younger than you are now? Can you imagine what you will feel like in 10 or 20 years' time? Do you expect to feel any different?

WHAT ARE ATTITUDES?

Attitudes can be defined as 'fixed modes of thinking'; everyone has a range of attitudes about all kinds of issues; about politics, lifestyles, food, architecture and people. Attitudes are formed throughout our lives, many being developed in our childhood. The major influences in attitude formation are the family, the school and one's peer group. Attitudes help people to be ready to react or respond in a predetermined way to a situation. They are important personality characteristics and help people form groupings (Hilgard, Atkinson and Atkinson 1971). It is apparent that our attitudes affect how people behave in everyday situations. Belief breeds behaviour. It is hard to see that it is possible to have consistently good practice if the staff have negative attitudes.

It is often said that attitudes can not be changed easily; this belief then excuses people from attempting to challenge and modify negative attitudes. Few individuals would be ready to admit that they have closed minds full of fixed beliefs; most people wish to think that they are open minded and ready to listen to new ideas. Trainers and managers must assume that attitudes are able to be changed and where negative attitudes persist despite training it may be more appropriate to reconsider the value and appropriateness of the training.

ATTITUDES TO OLD PEOPLE

No other section of the community is so vulnerable to being labelled and stereotyped. There seem to be two extremes: the sentimental 'Darby and Joan' image and the 'senile decrepit' (Brown 1982). 'The elderly' are seen as a 'bottomless pit' swallowing up the resources of health and social services which would be far better spent on prevention of illness and treatment of younger age groups (Norman 1982). None of us wish to die young. It therefore follows that we all wish to reach 'old age', however it is defined. In spite of this we still have a dread of old age and ageing. This means that older people form a unique 'minority' group that has many associated negative connotations but that most people aspire to join.

In our society, age is used as an important indicator of a person's legal rights and responsibilities and as a gauge of their likely position in life, their outlook and their activities (Garrett 1990). It is assumed that a teenager will be a devotee of 'heavy metal' music, be a late riser and like 'fast food'. Someone in their 40s will be at the zenith of their career, be settled and have given up some of the more energetic sports of their youth. Someone in their 80s will be arthritic, frightened of being mugged and intolerant of youth. Like all stereotypes there is a grain of truth in these statements, but some teenagers like classical music, some people in their 40s are just taking up a new career and some 80-year-olds are regularly running marathons. It could be argued that you are not old if you are still independent; if age is viewed in this way then the vast majority of the retired population is not old (Brown 1982). How individuals feel about their own old age is often a matter of their attitudes and beliefs and may be affected by lessons learned from their parents and grandparents. Many people in their 70s and 80s have a more youthful outlook than others in their 30s and 40s. For these people their actual age is irrelevant. Other people have grown up with a less positive view of age and their fears and horrors of old age become a self-fulfilling prophecy.

When 'old' is used as an adjective it can have two meanings. The first has a negative feel and implies that the object is past its best and has seen better days (old car, old clothes). The second meaning, which is more benevolent, hints at a feeling of warmth and familiarity and of a long-standing relationship (old friend, old teddy bear). When 'old' is applied to people it most often carries a negative connotation.

In common parlance in the western world, 'old' is taken to mean people over retirement age. Society does not attempt to clump together people aged 0 to 35 years old, yet finds it possible to include all 65- to 100-year-olds in a seemingly homogeneous group. The ages of 65–100 years can include people from at least two generations and people with a multitude of interests, abilities and experiences. One of the reasons for this device is that it neatly divides people who are no longer productive from those who are still productive. This simple device gave rise to the notion that 'old' people are a burden on the younger generation. The life span of most of the animal kingdom is related to the ability to procreate and the ability to 'work' by gathering food. People in the twentieth century can expect to live beyond this stage (Scrutton 1989), but there is no clear role for older people and the individual's experience of old age will depend on their place in the social structure (Estes 1986).

In earlier centuries people either worked until they were too frail to continue or until they had no financial need to work; recent history has invented both childhood and old age. This view of older people is not universal. In developing countries older people tend to have a continued useful role; they may not be productive but may take the roles of child-minders or teachers. The artificial grouping of older people, as seen in developed countries, has two dominant stereotypes. There is the stereotype of 'inevitability' that sees older people as dejected and rejected and the stereotype of 'tranquillity' that defines older people as 'contented, gracious and resigned' (Garrett 1990). Neither description is apposite; both of the word pictures can be applied to people of any age. There is the stereotype that sees all older people as needing assistance and the majority of older people being 'in care'. Yet the 1991 census information indicates that less than 6 per cent of people over retirement age are either in residential or nursing accommodation (OPCS 1991).

Language and labelling play an important part in discrimination. It is worth remembering that 'geriatric' is derived from the Greek and is an adjective that literally means 'treatment in old age'; thus there can be geriatric units but not geriatric people (Garrett 1990). Interestingly there is not such a temptation, it appears, to call a child a 'paediatric' or a pregnant woman an 'obstetric'.

Perversely, most older people do not often think of themselves as old until they are ill or unhappy (Marshall 1990a) but a number of people, as they age, will take note of current stereotypes and assume that they accurately describe their future. Ageism can be internalised by its victims who then share the stereotype and come to comply with the ageist society's expectations. This may mean that the future quality of life of some older people may be determined more by other people's expectations of them than by their own health and social situation.

If someone believes that illness is an inevitable part of growing old, they may have low expectations of any health care programme. Consider the number of older people who, on admission to hospital, appear to be suffering from a chronic urinary tract infection and who have never presented for treatment. If someone thinks that as an older person they should be resigned and not make a fuss, they will not usually complain about poor services or demand better services. An example of this would be the absence of complaints about the long waiting lists for some treatments used extensively by older people (e.g. chiropody, occupational therapy). Some older people too easily accept a prescribed social role which is limiting, inhibiting and unrewarding. These people then may suffer from a resulting lack of power and influence. Those older people who resist these stereotypes may be seen as 'rebellious', 'uncooperative' and 'difficult'. Older people who are labelled in this way run the subsequent risk of being labelled as eccentric or mentally ill. It is a classic 'no win' situation!

There is a trend for health to be defined in ways that are more helpful. While Freud wrote that old people were 'inflexible and ineducable' (Freud 1905) a more recent definition of health has been:

> the ability to adapt to changing environments, to growing and ageing, to healing when damaged, to suffering and to the peaceful expectation of death. (Illich 1977)

There is an idea often promulgated in both political and media circles that the population is rapidly becoming overwhelmed by the old and the 'very old' — hence the use of such a phrase as 'the rising tide'. There will be a growth in the numbers of older people during the next few years but the proportion of the population who are retired is remarkably similar now to that of nearly 30 years ago. In 1965, 12.2 per cent of the population was retired; by 1975 the figure had risen to 14.1 per cent and to 14.7 per cent in 1985. In 1995 it is estimated that the proportion will have dropped to 14.4 per cent (OPCS 1991).

Professionals involved in the provision of caring services often describe older people as 'lonely' and many day centres see one of their aims as being the relief of loneliness. While the 1991 census did show that 25 per cent of retired people live alone, two things must be remembered: first, that many live alone by choice and not by necessity and secondly, that being alone is not the same as being lonely. Even where older people describe themselves as 'lonely', it may be entirely inappropriate to imagine that encouraging them to spend 5 or 6 hours in the company of strangers in an unfamiliar day centre will solve their problem. Of course, a proportion of people attending day centres do get to know other people, building meaningful relationships, but many will find the prospect daunting and will refuse the service offered. Others will visit once or twice and decide that 'they do not fit in'.

It must not be forgotten that people can suffer from more than one form of discrimination at a time. Substantial problems are being faced by some older people from ethnic minorities. They were discriminated against throughout their working life, often taking menial jobs with poor wages and with no opportunity to invest in a pension plan. They may have lived in substandard housing and been educationally disadvantaged (Marshall 1990b). In old age they may find themselves discovering that support services are neither easily accessible to them nor tailored to their needs. Their problems are eloquently described as the 'triple jeopardy' by Alison Norman (Norman 1985). Older people from ethnic minorities are also particularly vulnerable to physical and mental illness (Hughes and Bhaduri 1987). Professionals must ensure that they are familiar with the culture and aware of the stereotypes that may relate to different situations. It is easy to assume, for example, that all Asian families will look after their elders and to see the low referral rate from this group as support for this hypothesis. Staff must be aware that a low referral rate can equally be a reflection of the inaccessibility of a service, the lack of publicity material in appropriate languages or the general lack of credibility of a service among potential ethnic users.

ATTITUDES TO SERVICES FOR OLDER PEOPLE – THE 'CINDERELLA' SERVICES

It is widely believed that social work with older people is less challenging than work with children. Certainly there is less statutory work. It could be argued that working without the benefit and guidance of a framework of law makes working with older people more challenging, requiring the worker to be more confident and more skilled. Some techniques, such as counselling and family therapy, are rarely used with older people. Why? Is it because there is an assumption that the needs of older people are simple, easily assessed and easily satisfied (Scrutton 1989)? A large proportion of every social work department's budget is spent on older people yet there are still few qualified social workers employed to work specifically with older people. Social work training, like medicine, has not focused in the past on the potential of working with older people (Murphy 1986).

Within the nursing profession similar views are still held; the notion of the 'back ward' and the lack of status of 'geriatric nursing' are still current. Nurses are still told to work in the acute sector if they 'wish to get on'. Health visitors have a remit to provide a service to older people, but workload pressures usually mean that they spend most or all of their time working with children and families. Things have begun to change, with special interest groups now existing within both the Royal College of Nursing and the British Association of Social Workers.

The medical profession has also not escaped from this prejudice. Some doctors see geriatric medicine as a second-rate speciality, looking after third-rate patients in fourth-rate facilities (BMA 1986). This prejudice is held in spite of the fact that at any one moment in time a large number of NHS beds are filled with people over 65 years old. Those professionals who already work with older people know that the work can provide opportunities to work with an exceptional and interesting group of adults (Marshall 1990c). There are opportunities to work with colleagues from other agencies and to use a wide range of interventions. Unfortunately, all too often staff are the culprits of ageist practice, colluding to provide a second-rate service. Some talented staff, in choosing to work with older people, know that they will have diminished their career opportunities.

Care staff working with older people in residential units, by the very nature of their work, see the most frail older people, often coming to believe that all old people are in the same condition. They usually have few role models of positive ageing. The situation is little better among those staff based in the community.

There is a dilemma in the continual need to emphasise the range and extent of the problems faced by those older people who are the most vulnerable and frail, while still emphasising the talents, skills and good health of the majority. However, things are changing. The last few years have seen the development of numerous courses focusing on the care of older people and the studying of gerontology has become more respected as a challenging and rigorous academic pursuit. The establishment of Nursing Development Units in units caring for older people has led to innovative practice. In many areas social service departments have re-examined the services offered to older people and have developed more appropriate ways of providing care to people who are older. The full implementation of the NHS and Community Care Act should provide further incentives for the development of creative responses by the statutory, voluntary and private sectors.

In addition, there has been a recognition in recent years of the existence of the problem of the abuse of vulnerable adults. The government has provided guidelines for dealing with such abuse and individual statutory authorities have prepared guidelines for staff and in most cases have appreciated that the best basis for these guidelines are those established in child care.

Quality Assurance initiatives and inspection have been developed that encourage positive practice and the power of the carers' lobby has ensured that poor care is no longer acceptable. Carers have, with their increased self-confidence, demanded more of the services both for the person they care for and for themselves. Psychological and counselling skills now have a much higher profile in helping people to see the benefit of appropriately qualified and skilled staff.

ATTITUDES TO MENTAL ILLNESS IN OLDER PEOPLE

There is a widespread belief that psychiatric illnesses are an intrinsic part of ageing (Buckwater, Smith and Martin 1993). Even where it is recognised that this is not the case, symptoms are still often described as diagnoses, e.g. 'confused' and 'senile' (Norman 1982). Most people, if asked to name a mental illness found in older people, will think of dementia, forgetting that older people can suffer from all of the psychiatric disorders found in those under retirement age. Older people are not immune to depression, anxiety or phobic states. Many older people are condemned to live (and die) with treatable and alleviable illnesses and unidentified sensory deficits.

There is still a substantial degree of difference in the status of those who care for people with functional illnesses and those who care for people with dementia. Care professionals like to see a 'cure' at the end of a course of 'treatment'.

> We like to see people getting better or if they must die, in a tidy way so that we can demonstrate our terminal care skills. (Brown 1982)

The care of older people with dementia is not like that: people with dementia can appear frightening and ungrateful and their needs can rarely be packaged 'neatly'. Equally in dementia care there is an erroneous belief that there is little scope for therapeutic interventions. In fact, the care of people with moderate dementia and a degree of insight into their problem calls for skilled interventions, while the care of profoundly demented people needs imaginative responses and supportive strategies (Levin, Sinclair and Gorbach 1983). Oliver (1983) described a social model of disability that suggests that any disability should be seen not only as the result of an impairment of an individual but also as society's inability to make plans to accommodate people who are not fit in body and mind. It is not the fault of older people that they are lonely, in pain or isolated. Their situation is not a result of bad decisions nor of ineffective coping mechanisms, but a result of the lack of appropriate resources and ancillary services. This model also applies to dementia care. The 'solutions' available to assist someone who has dementia have been both primitive and scarce and rarely tailored to meet the person's individual needs.

Ten years ago most areas would have had a psychogeriatric unit headed by a psychogeriatrician. Recent years have seen a renaming of many of these units to Departments for the Mental Health of Older People headed by a 'psychiatrist of old age'. These changes are more than cosmetic; they indicate a greater interest in a positive approach, an emphasis on health promotion and a desire to shed unhelpful labels. Similarly (and fortunately) the use of the term EMI (Elderly Mentally Infirm) seems to be diminishing.

The care of older people with mental health problems should be seen as a rewarding area of professional practice, with an appropriate theoretical framework and conceptual base.

ATTITUDES OF PROFESSIONALS TO EACH OTHER

In the recent past numerous multidisciplinary teams have been established and operated with varying degrees of success. The NHS and Community Care Act 1990 has focused minds on the provision of community-based services and the design, implementation and delivery of these services are often dependent on the ability of staff from different agencies to work together. The 1990 Act has extended the range of people with whom staff from the statutory agencies need to develop working relationships and there is now a need to establish and nurture effective working relationships with both the private and voluntary sectors.

The effectiveness of relationships between staff from different backgrounds will be affected by the attitudes and stereotypes that one group believes of the other. It is worth looking closer at some of these stereotypes and beliefs and attempting to identify how they may hinder effective working partnerships. Does it matter that nurses think all social workers wear sandals and drive small French cars? Does it matter that social workers think that nurses all prefer to wear a uniform and are preoccupied with pills, potions and bowels? On one level these beliefs are amusing and harmless, but they often disguise a lack of knowledge and understanding about each professional's value base, interest and code of conduct.

Wherever possible groups of staff who are trying to provide an integrated service should put aside time to 'get to know each other' and come to an understanding about the way each agency operates. Nurses and medical staff often do not appreciate the ramifications that result from Social Services departments having political masters at County Council level. Equally, social workers are not always aware of the impact of having a system of professional accountability and registration.

The private and voluntary sectors have suffered from prejudice from staff in both statutory agencies; too often proprietors of private residential or nursing homes have been labelled as being solely orientated to maximising profit. As a result they have often not been treated as colleagues in the 'planning of care' process and their views not invited nor treated as having equal weight. Staff in statutory agencies need to be aware that they 'make money' out of caring for older people and that there is as much variety of experience and motivation in the statutory and private sectors.

No one is exempt from negative attitudes. Many people would tell you that GPs are always rushed, employ obstructive receptionists and rarely do house calls; that hospital staff are more concerned with bed clearing than how someone will manage at home; that wardens in sheltered housing only check that residents are 'alive' and that home helps do not clean windows or hang curtains.

Staff from different agencies will only be able to gain an insight into each other's work if they are given time to do so. Consideration should be given to the possibility of job swaps and shadowing in order to facilitate increased understanding and effective networking.

ATTITUDES TO CARERS

Misconceptions about people apply to carers just as much as to professionals. Each carer will have their own attitudes to professional care givers that will reflect many of the attitudes already described. Perhaps of more importance are the attitudes and stereotypes that professionals hold of carers. Some staff seem to spend time and effort identifying an individual patient's or resident's needs and drawing up a personalised 'care plan' only to make crude assumptions about what their carer will need, want and prefer. Carers are as diverse in their interests, tolerance and fortitude as anyone else; they have different breaking points and different coping strategies. It is as unhelpful to believe that all carers are wonderful people as to believe that all carers abuse the person they care for. Professional care staff must not assume that the problems they perceive in the care of someone with dementia will be the same as the carer's view. An example of this would be the desire of hospital staff to increase someone's mobility, not appreciating that the carer may find someone who is less mobile, and therefore less inclined to wander, easier to care for. This is not to imply that the carer is always right or can always dictate the style of care or the appropriateness of treatment. Equally, it is not the case that staff can ignore the carer's perspective if the object is to maintain, at home, the person with dementia.

Ethical dilemmas such as this are common in the care of people with dementia. There is no simple, single answer but each team of care staff needs to have the time, space and structure that will allow the discussion of each issue and the attempt to find a resolution (Fairbairn and Mead 1993).

ATTITUDES OF OLDER PEOPLE TO CARE

The attitudes of older people themselves to care is an important issue. The generation that is now in their 80s were not brought up to be 'consumer' orientated; most of these older people will remember life before the welfare state and may find the notions of empowerment, advocacy and complaint systems unfamiliar. Many professionals report a reluctance among some older people to complain about the service they are offered, often being grateful for whatever they receive, no matter what its quality. There are more older women in care and receiving community support; women of this generation are more likely to be submissive (Stevenson 1989). Consider, for example, the person who dislikes the meals offered by her local Meals on Wheels service but takes the dinners, feeding them to her cat because she does not want to upset anyone, or the case of an older person who waits until a medical problem becomes unbearable because they did not want to bother the GP.

Staff need to find ways of reminding people that they have paid, or are paying, for the services they receive and as such have a right and a duty to express their opinion of the service. If they are reluctant to do it for themselves they may be persuaded to comment for the sake of those who will follow.

VALUES

The King's Fund publication *Living Well into Old Age* (1986) provided professional care staff with a set of values that should serve as the basis for any service. They are quoted in full.

- People with dementia have the same human value as anyone else irrespective of their degree of disability or dependence.
- People with dementia have the same varied human needs as anyone else.
- People with dementia have the same rights as other citizens.
- Every person with dementia is an individual.
- People with dementia have the right to forms of support which do not exploit family and friends.

The vast majority of staff involved in the care of people with dementia will agree with these values. If staff are involved in discussions about a resuscitation policy for people with dementia, or considering 'tagging' as a safety device, or deciding whether to involve users of the service in review meetings, they should consider how they will reconcile their decision with these values.

FINANCES AND RATIONING

Older people experience a wide range of financial conditions; many older people exist on state benefits but an increasing number are eligible for occupational pensions, making their financial position more assured. Many older people are asset-rich, i.e. they own a house, but income-poor. Others are poorly advised by professionals, trying to live on the interest their savings attract while saving their capital for a 'rainy day'. The greatest fear of many old people remains 'being a burden'. Older people who have money will have more choice in the services they use and they will not be affected by the strictures of the Social Services community care budgets and eligibility criteria.

Government policy seems to be designed to bring about financial dependency in older people. The National Health Service and Community Care Act (1990) was introduced mainly to staunch the flow of Social Security money being spent on residential and nursing care. There is a great imperative for all providers of health care to unit cost each service they provide. One can imagine that some health commissioners may have to decide, at some point in the future, not to fund expensive procedures for older people, given that it is more difficult to prove 'value for money'. The numbers of continuing care beds provided by Health Authorities is continually decreasing, with large numbers of these beds being 'contracted out' to the private sector. The rationale for this is mainly one of saving money. If this is the case why are acute beds never 'contracted out'?

The benefits system is notoriously complex; a range of issues affect older people's ability to claim appropriate benefits. Older people may perceive some benefits as 'charity': some people aged 80 years and over will have a memory of the workhouse and the associated Poor Law. Some older people will be unaware of their eligibility for benefits with many people, including professionals, believing that one can only claim the Attendance Allowance if one lives alone. The initiative to claim benefits lies with the older person and their carers; they may have difficulty finding the time and energy to obtain and complete the relevant forms. Every unit offering care to older people should ensure that a member of staff is either familiar with the benefit system or knows how to access skilled advice.

THE LEGAL POSITION

The legal position of older people is, in most respects, the same as the position of all adults. This could be because society is non-ageist, and has chosen not to distinguish between people's needs for legal protection on the basis of age. It is more likely that older people have not been represented in the powerful lobbies in society that affect the shape of our laws. This is illustrated by the way the law copes with abuse. It could be argued that all abuse can be dealt with by recourse to the criminal laws covering actual bodily harm, assault and fraud. Society has deemed it appropriate to create structures and procedures that relate particularly to the abuse of children because they have a special vulnerability. Society has not chosen to design similar procedures to cope with the abuse of vulnerable older people. Fortunately, the problem is being partially addressed. Over the last few years guidelines have been developed in many Health and Social Services areas. The gap in any of these systems is the absence of the equivalent of a 'Place of Safety' order for vulnerable adults.

Care staff need to have an understanding of the laws that affect older people (Power of Attorney, Court of Protection orders, Mental Health Act, Section 47 of the National Assistance Act 1948, etc.). They also need to be aware of professionally qualified people in their area who are interested, willing and well informed and who are prepared to give sound advice to older people and their carers (Age Concern 1986).

There are several ways in which older people with mental health problems are affected either by the lack of law or by misapplication of the law. Often there is a reluctance to apply the Mental Health Act to older people with dementia. They may urgently need admission to hospital but refuse the offer of a bed. Rather than apply the appropriate section of the Act some workers think it less damaging to 'persuade' the older person to go into hospital; this might be through continued pressure or by literally 'taking the older person for a ride'. Even if the older person settles into hospital they remain voluntary patients, usually without the means to seek their own discharge. If the Mental Health Act had been applied to them they would have had the protection of the appeals procedure and the overview of the Mental Health Commission (Marshall 1990a).

SEXUALITY

Many of the textbooks written about the care of older people do not address issues of sexuality. For a variety of reasons there is a belief that older people 'do not do it'. This may have arisen because of the direct relationship between sexual activity and reproduction: when the opportunity for procreation has passed, sexual activity becomes tainted with thoughts of inappropriateness. In fact, 60 per cent of couples remain sexually active into their mid and late 70s (Brown 1982).

Consider the expression 'dirty old man'; how has this saying entered our language when all the statistics indicate that most sexual offences are perpetrated by men in their 20s and 30s? If the belief that most people over retirement age are not sexually active is current, then it is hardly surprising that an extension of the belief is that people with dementia should not be sexually active. In the vocabulary of care 'inappropriate behaviour' has become a euphemism for overt sexual activity in people with dementia. Professional care staff are often diligent when trying to identify stresses for carers yet few invite carers to identify problems associated with either the lack of a sexual element in the relationship or an unacceptable change in the previous pattern of sexual activity. Carers may be concerned because they have continued sexual feelings to their partner, but are reluctant to express these feelings when their partner may not always recognise them. Some carers may have feelings approaching revulsion at the thought of maintaining a sexual relationship with a demented partner.

Care staff should also be sensitive to the range of sexual relationships that older people may have had. Older people are just as likely as younger people to have formed homosexual or lesbian partnerships, yet these relationships are often dismissed or ignored by care staff. At its most extreme it can mean that homosexual partners of 30 or 40 years' standing can not even be counted as 'next of kin' and may be denied access or influence in a variety of planning processes.

Care professionals should be able to make provision within all residential units for privacy and should ensure that issues relating to sexuality are considered in the care planning process. Consideration should be given to having a member of staff trained to offer advice on sexual matters in the same way that staff may take a special interest in continence, AIDS and reminiscence therapy.

RIGHTS VERSUS RISKS

The rights of a person with dementia are exactly the same as any other person suffering with any mental illness, with rights enshrined in the Mental Health Act 1983. Until a person is deemed to be mentally incompetent by a doctor they should be consulted on all aspects of care.

Most of the care provided either within the bureaucracies of Social Services or the Health Authority occurs within a framework of rules that exist to minimise the risks, minimise the possibility of litigations and to conform to the general public's expectation that these bodies should act responsibly and keep people 'safe'. An over-preoccupation with safety will usually minimise older people's rights and choices. This argument has been used in past years to justify the locking of doors on wards for older people with dementia and more recently consideration of electronic tagging schemes.

Public opinion about safety may also influence the style of domiciliary care provision. Take the situation of an older person with dementia, living at home in some degree of squalor: the home help service has been requested to offer support; the older person is reluctant to let anyone in the house and denies vehemently that they are unable to cope. Over the next few weeks the domestic situation deteriorates but the home helps succeed in gaining the older person's trust and are now regularly allowed into the sitting room. Neighbours may find the situation and the slowness of the intervention hard to bear. They may complain of the emotive risks of infestations and fire hazards. In many cases, before the helping agencies can be in a position to affect the situation the neighbourhood has decided that they can tolerate no more. A rash of telephone calls and visits to various officials will often result in the older person being admitted to care 'for their own safety'. The 'something must be done' syndrome is widespread. Unfortunately a person's right to live at home for as long as they wish is affected by the location of their home; the person who lives in a detached house in a rural setting will be allowed to live in a more high-risk situation than the person who lives in a house of multi-occupation.

SELF AWARENESS OF STAFF

All therapeutic relationships are based on the ability of people to empathise with one another (Stevenson 1989). Staff who work with older people will not have had the experiences that old people have had. The gap between their experiences is often wide, particularly if one considers those older people who have lived through two world wars. Many staff will have had experience of bereavement but may not have had to face the multiple bereavements that older people face as their family and social circle shrink. It could be hypothesised that older people deal with bereavements in a different way to younger people and that this difference relates to the realisation of their own mortality.

Staff may not have personally experienced organic illness and even those staff who have sensitively cared for people with dementia for many years may have found ways of distancing themselves from the pain of the possibility that they may suffer from the disease. Staff should be committed to providing care to a standard that would be acceptable to themselves.

Where younger people are caring for people older than themselves there is a risk that the older people will be invested with some of the negative characteristics of unliked and unloved older people from the past. Unresolved attitudes to parents, grandparents and teachers may obstruct the development of helpful relationships.

Care professionals also need to think for themselves about the feelings associated with forced dependency. What is it like not to be in control? Many younger people will only have experienced this if they have spent a period of time in hospital, where the needs of the organisation may have caused a loss of dignity, individuality and choice in spite of good, modern nursing practice. People who provide care are often upset if the people they provide care for do not express gratitude. It is helpful occasionally to imagine what it would be like if one is dependent and has to say 'thank you' and be grateful when staff undertake those mundane tasks that everyone else takes for granted. Every expression of gratitude emphasises the dependency.

Most older people with dementia become dependent and yet by the very nature of the illness they may not only not be sufficiently grateful but may be actually hostile. The quantity and quality of hostility can sometimes be altered if staff do not expect to be thanked and provide each episode of practical care giving in a low key manner, seeking permission to assist wherever possible.

Staff who are new to working with older people may find it incongruous being 'responsible' for a group of people who are old enough to be their parents or grandparents. There needs to be acknowledgement of the power relationships and group dynamics and a realisation that most older people have few options about the care they receive. They can often not object, may have no real choice about the kind of provision and can not escape from the inevitability of needing help in many areas of daily life.

ACTION FOR CHANGE

1. Get the staff group to describe/draw a typical nurse, social worker, doctor, old person. What similarities are there in the images described

or drawn by different team members? Do they have any relationship to real people?

2. Managers and supervisors should spend time in supervision talking to staff about their hopes for their old age, talking to staff about their experiences of ageing and helping them relate these experiences to their current beliefs and practices.

3. Examine the language used in the unit. Do people talk or write about 'the elderly'? Is the term EMI in use? Is there talk of people suffering from dementia? Do staff think they know what terms are preferred by older people and their carers? Consider raising the issue of terminology in a carers' meeting.

4. Collect material that relates to older people who are enjoying retirement and finding it a time of opportunity. Find ways in which staff can be involved with 'normal healthy' older people. Could staff be involved in health promotion activities locally?

5. Examine some of the routines of the unit. Are they based on negative attitudes? For example, review the practice of making up a bed for a new resident. Are incontinence pads or draw sheets used automatically?

6. Get each member of the staff team to sit back and look at the service your unit offers. Ask if they would allow their parents/grandparents to use the service? If not, what would need to change to make the service acceptable? Discuss these changes. What stops them happening?

7. Review the process associated with the formulation of a care plan. On what basis are the targets/goals set? Is the carer consulted about the expectations? Are the expectations usually over-ambitious or not?

8. How do you decide what activities and outings to arrange? Are you basing your choice on the staff's view of what is interesting and appropriate? What would fit, healthy older people living nearby suggest?

REFERENCES

Age Concern (1986) *The Law and Vulnerable Elderly People*. London: Age Concern.

British Medical Association (1986) *All Our Tomorrows: Growing Old in Britain*. Report of the BMA's Board of Science and Education. London: British Medical Association.

Brown P (1982) *The Other Side of Growing Old*. London: Macmillan.

Buckwater K, Smith M and Martin M (1993) Attitude problem. *Nursing Times* 89(5): 55–57.

Estes C L (1986) The politics of ageing in America. *Aging and Society* 6(2): 121–34.

Fairbairn G and Mead D (1993) Working with stories nurses tell. *Nursing Standard* 7(31): 37–40.

Freud S (1905) *On Psychotherapy*. London: Hogarth Press.

Garrett G (1990) *Older People. Their Support and Care.* London: Macmillan.

Hilgard E, Atkinson R and Atkinson R (1971) *Introduction to Psychology,* 5th edn. New York: Harcourt Brace Jovanovich.

Hughes R D and Bhaduri R (1987) *Race and Culture in Service Delivery.* London: DHSS.

Illich I (1977) *Limits to Medicine.* Harmondsworth: Pelican.

King's Fund Centre Project Paper No 23 (1986) *Living Well into Old Age.* London: King's Fund Publishing Office.

Levin E, Sinclair I and Gorbach P (1983) *The Supporters of Confused Persons at Home.* London: Macmillan.

Marshall M (1990a) *Social Work with Older People,* 2nd edn. London: Macmillan.

Marshall M (1990b) Proud to be Old. Attitudes to Age and Ageing. In: McEwen E (ed.) *Age. The Unrecognised Discrimination. Views to Provoke a Debate.* London: Age Concern.

Marshall M (1990c) *Working with Dementia. Guidelines for Professionals.* Birmingham: Venture Press.

Mental Health Act (1983) London: DSS.

Murphy E (1986) *Dementia and Mental Illness in the Old.* London: Papermac.

National Health Service and Community Care Act (1990) London: HMSO.

Norman A (1982) *Mental Illness in Old Age: Meeting the Challenge.* London: Centre for Policy on Ageing.

Norman A (1985) *Triple Jeopardy: Growing Old in a Second Homeland.* London: Centre for Policy on Ageing.

Office of Population Censuses and Surveys (1991) *Preliminary Report for England and Wales.* London: HMSO.

Oliver M (1983) *Social Work with Disabled People.* London: British Association of Social Workers, Macmillan.

Scrutton S (1989) *Counselling Older People. A Creative Response to Aging. Age Concern Handbook.* London: Edward Arnold.

Stevenson O (1989) *Age and Vulnerability A Guide to Better Care. Age Concern Handbook.* London: Edward Arnold.

2 Getting Old
Establishing what is normal 'ageing'

In order to understand the problems of dementia in older people it is necessary first to be able to appreciate what can be considered as the normal ageing process. Dementia may affect up to 5 per cent of older people aged over 65 years and 20 per cent of those over the age of 80 years. Restated, this means that 95 per cent of people over the age of 65 do not have dementia, along with 80 per cent of people over 80 years old (Hofman, Roca and Brayne 1991).

If professionals have no conception about the range of experiences and changes faced by people as they age normally they cannot begin to identify abnormality. It is possible that staff constantly working with ill health often have a distorted image of what is the norm for older people and what can be achieved.

POINTS TO PONDER

- The last time you forgot a message did you apologise and blame it on a poor memory due to age?

- Do you think that the reason older people find difficulty in using computers is because they have a lower IQ than younger people?

- All older people have bowel problems because bowel control deteriorates with age. Do you agree with this statement?

- What do you consider to be the normal sleep requirement for a person aged 75 years?

- Do you feel that older people have the need for a political voice of their own?

- What is the temperature of your unit? Is there a reason for this?

- How many older people that you know live within 2 miles of their children?

• Is it right that some large companies adopt a policy of employing newly retired people when there is so much unemployment?

WHAT IS NORMAL AGEING?

The only thing that people can be sure of in this life is that they will die. What disease or accident will cause death and the way a person will age cannot be predicted. Ageing does not start at 65, everybody is getting older; today we are older than yesterday, and there is always somebody younger than you. So what is normal ageing? Is it normal to be grey-haired and arthritic at 50, 60 or 70 years?

It is very rare that an adult survives to the age of 70 or 80 years without having some disease process affecting their body, so to separate normal ageing from pathological ageing may be misleading; it is felt by some to be a mere academic exercise (Bromley 1988). It is acknowledged that there are changes in the organs and biochemistry of the human body that are consistent with people who are in the third age of their life. Changes are also noted in activity and process (Bromley 1988) which will be discussed later in the chapter. Old age is described by Bromley, rather harshly but briefly, as:

> human ageing can be conveniently defined as a complex, cumulative, time-related process of psychological deterioration occupying the post-developmental (adult) phase of life.

The human life path, commencing at conception, leading through childhood, adolescence, adulthood to old age describes the chronological development of a person. However, when someone stops being an adult and starts being old is less clear. The 'young old' aged 65 years who are newly retired are manifestly different from the 'old old', who are normally deemed to be over 85 years. From 85 years onwards the 'old old' person becomes more physically and mentally disabled until the breakdown of their body ends in death. So why do some people appear to age quicker that others? Why is chronological age no longer an accurate yardstick by which to judge a person's abilities?

BIOLOGICAL THEORIES OF AGEING

There are a number of theories of ageing and it is commonly accepted by biologists that ageing has a molecular basis which manifests as deterioration and alteration in cellular and organ behaviour (Warnes 1989).

To describe the several main theories in depth would not be appropriate but to understand basic concepts of ageing in simple terms may, in turn, lead to a clearer overview of the ageing process.

The theories are based on the idea that normal physiological activity alters in old age; for example, the Somatic Mutation theory states that as people age there is more likelihood of DNA replicating incorrectly or failing to replicate at all. Other theories are based on the notion that there is additional or new physiological activity in old age. These theories would include the Free Radical theory, which is based on the concept that 'free radicals', which are electrically charged chemicals, attract excess waste from oxygen metabolism. This in turn reacts with DNA proteins and lipids thereby causing defects in the replication of cells. It would also include the Cross-linkage theory which hypothesises that additional linkages are formed between proteins, making them change their normal character and affecting the way they function.

Other theories have a more fatalistic approach; the Programmed Ageing theory speculates that ageing is a preprogrammed process in the DNA and the Wear and Tear theory states that the body's structures and functions wear out or are over-used (Ebersole and Hess 1985; Warnes 1989).

NON-BIOLOGICAL THEORIES OF AGEING

Alongside these biological theories of ageing there are a range of psychological, social and evolutionary theories which are more philosophical in nature (Ebersole and Hess 1985). The 'Evolutionary' theory holds that old age has simply evolved as an addendum to the life of sexual maturation and propagation; the theory is supported by Jung, Erikson and Clayton, who state that old age is a time provided for reflection, wisdom and a vantage point to look back at one's life.

Sociologists view old age as a time regulated and stifled by arbitrary age restrictions and stereotypes. This leads to people having lowered expectations of life and fewer opportunities for older people to fulfil their potential.

HOW LONG WILL WE LIVE?

The longevity of man has risen from an average of 47 years to 73 years this century, mainly due to improved living conditions and the decrease in disease. In 1951 in the UK the Queen sent 271 messages of congratulation to people celebrating their 100th birthdays. In 1981 she sent 2410 (Coni, Davison and Webster 1992). Yet to live longer does not necessarily mean an improved quality of life. The statistics of ageing are a poor indicator of the quality of life that people experience; for example, statistics show that the proportion of people in care rises with age but this provides little information about how satisfied these older people are with their lives.

PHYSICAL AGEING

The ageing process is a collection of phenomena that interrelate to produce an individual response in each person. For simplicity each of these processes will be examined in isolation. Many care professionals will have firm ideas about how different systems and processes are affected by age; some of these ideas are partial truths and some are based on myths and 'old wives' tales'. It is helpful to try to establish what is generally true and what is misleading, but commonly held, fallacy in order to have an accurate picture of what is normal in old age and what may relate to the presence of dementia.

The Digestive System

The Allegation

'Constipation is normal in all older people'.

The Evidence

The digestive system stretches from the mouth to the anus; there are changes in the system as people age, commencing at the mouth with a decline in the sense of taste and a decrease in the secretion of saliva. There are also disturbances in normal peristalsis within the intestinal tract and stomach (Bromley 1988), impairment of absorption from the small intestine and a reduction in acid secreted due to atrophy of the gastric mucosa. There is also a change in the flora of the large bowel and an increase in the time it takes for material to pass through the large bowel. These changes can cause a tendency to constipation (Roberts 1987).

Summing Up

Many professionals who work with older people expect them to have a bowel problem and it is accepted as a normal part of the ageing process.

This is true in part but the main cause of constipation in the elderly is the ritualistic purgation with laxatives that used to occur with children in the 1920s and 1930s. A cathartic colon is an exaggerated response to constraint and chronic purgative treatment and some patients, once addicted, are never able to recover satisfactorily (Roberts 1987). The most damaging aperients with prolonged use include Liquid Paraffin and 'health salts' which may cause electrolyte disturbance (BNF 1993).

Constipation is not 'normal', but a tendency to constipation may occur in some older people; it is often compounded by laxative abuse and poor diet.

The Renal System

The Allegation

Most older people are incontinent and appropriate aids and furnishings should always be available.

The Evidence

The kidney has been identified as an organ that deteriorates with age. It has been calculated that there is a reduction of 50 per cent efficiency between the ages of 30 and 60 years. The kidney shrinks, renal blood flow is reduced and the numbers of glomeruli halved (Roberts 1989b). These factors in turn cause an increase in the acid load, a potassium and sodium imbalance and a tendency for the kidneys to prevent excretion of drugs which may cause toxic effects. The damage due to longevity can be compounded by arteriosclerosis or high blood pressure (Coni, Davison and Webster 1992).

Bacteriuria becomes more common with old age with, on average, one in five people experiencing asymptomatic urinary tract infections. This is mainly due to the incomplete voidance of the bladder, or because of a decline in the immune system of the older person.

Problems with continence occur in 7 per cent of men and 12 per cent of women due to deterioration of muscle tone and nerve damage of various types (Van der Cammen, Rai and Exton-Smith 1991). It is, however, more often as a consequence of another disease process.

Summing Up

Evidence clearly shows that there is a decline in the efficiency of the renal system as people age with a higher probability that people have urinary tract infections. This does not mean that older people are inevitably going to be incontinent, but it will mean that most older people experience a change in the pattern of micturition.

Most people are not incontinent. Only one person in 10 has a continence problem and many of these problems can be rectified or ameliorated with assessment and treatment.

Vision, Hearing and Taste

The Allegation

Wearing glasses is a sign of old age; older people do not hear well, and they have a deteriorated sense of taste.

The Evidence

When the Queen began wearing glasses to read her speeches it was momentarily headline news, accepted as a sign of advancing years. Reading glasses are more common among older people as the lens of the eyes stretches and loses its ability to focus on near objects. The retina and ophthalmic pathway lose some of their cells making it harder to see detail and contrast (Warnes 1989); in addition colour discrimination and the ability to focus at dusk becomes more difficult (Coni, Davison and Webster 1992).

Hearing deteriorates and higher pitched sounds are harder to identify; however, the cause of this is unclear. The only obvious structural change in the ear is the atrophy of nervous tissue. There is, however, evidence that age does impair the ability of the person to interpret auditory information as quickly as younger people (Bromley 1988).

A person's ability to differentiate tastes does become affected by age, as the mucosa may become thicker and the number of taste buds reduce in the tongue (Roberts 1986).

Summing Up

The eyes and ears do deteriorate and taste becomes less sensitive. It is a normal sign of ageing.

The Cardiovascular System

The Allegation

Older people suffer from high blood pressure as the heart's pumping action becomes less effective.

The Evidence

The normal heart beats, on average, 72 times every minute; this equals an average of 103 680 times every 24 hours. Therefore, logically, it should be anticipated that age will affect this pump system, as with age there is a fall in the maximum heart rate achievable on exercise. There is also decreased contractivity in the heart and this causes a fall in cardiac output (Roberts 1988a). Because of the loss of elasticity in the arterial vascular system this causes blood pressure to rise even with decreased output (Coni, Davison and Webster 1992).

Summing Up

Blood pressure does increase with age in industrialised society. When an older person becomes clinically hypertensive, however, is difficult to define. The World Health Organisation defines hypertension in older people to be when the pressure is greater than 160/95 mmHg. Clinically, high blood pressure is not normal in old age (Van der Cammen et al 1991).

Respiratory System

The Allegation

Pneumonia is the 'old man's friend', in that it is the most likely cause of death.

The Evidence

It is very difficult to identify what a 'normal' lung and respiratory system is like in an older person because of the impact of external factors. The current population of older people was young and active in the 1930s, 1940s and 1950s when air pollution and smoking were the accepted norm. Diseased pathology therefore dominates older people; however, Roberts feels that true ageing probably affects gas exchange and there is less elasticity in the alveoli and the capillaries causing a degree of breathlessness as the norm (Van der Cammen et al 1991).

Summing Up

The 'normal' ageing lung has not been clearly identified, but older people do have an impaired functioning of their respiratory tract and are thus more likely to get chest infections, but it will not automatically cause death.

Activity, Mobility and the Skeletal System

The Allegation

If you keep fit when you are young it will stop you losing your muscle tone when you become older.

The Evidence

When somebody is becoming older the skeletal system and the muscles that support them often provide the visual evidence of ageing having occurred. Muscle strength declines and so lines and wrinkles occur. Within the muscle there is a slowing of collagen synthesis and so stamina decreases. Muscles contract if they are not used regularly, or if they are not able to be used because of disease (Roberts 1988b).

Bone mass is also lost with age and anecdotal stories of people shrinking with age may well be true, particularly in women, who tend to suffer from osteoporosis after the menopause due to a reduction in oestrogen production. Specific areas of bone mass, namely the joints, suffer damage through age, particularly the weight-bearing joints which develop thickening cartilage, less elasticity and some calcification (Roberts 1989b).

There is no evidence that participating in physical training will extend life expectancy, but it might increase the ability to resist disease or illness (Bromley 1988). Competitive sport could, some may argue, advance the ageing process by overstretching the body's abilities and producing 'burn out'. Young tennis stars are perhaps a common example of this.

Summing Up

Being very fit when you are young does not guarantee fitness in old age.

Homeostasis

The Allegation

Old people are vulnerable to death from hypothermia.

The Evidence

To a complementary therapist this term means being in a dynamic state of balance, to be together and centred (Norman 1989). It is technically described as a process where physiological mechanisms regulate and stabilise the internal environment. The ability of the body to redress the effect of exercise, the metabolism of glucose or regulating the body temperature becomes harder as the body becomes older. Homeostasis is less efficient in older people and so they are predisposed to problems such as late onset diabetes and hypothermia, because the body does not have the reserves that a younger person has (Bromley 1988).

Summing Up

All old people are vulnerable to hypothermia.

Sleep

The Allegation

Older people need less sleep than younger people.

The Evidence

The amount of sleep required by people varies from person to person, but there appears to be a norm of between 5.5 and 9.5 hours for adults. Older people require a little less, on average: about 6.5 hours. However, they experience altered sleep cycles, with more light sleep, of a poorer quality. They may also be awakened more easily in the middle of the night by noise and from discomfort with arthritic joints. They may need to get up to use the toilet and may have had frequent naps during the day (McMahon 1992). Women, even in old age, appear to enjoy a better quality of sleep than men (McMahon 1992).

Summing Up

Older people need less sleep than younger people in a 24-hour period; the pattern and quality of sleep may also change as people age.

Sexual Activity

The Allegation

Older people are not interested in sex and lack sex drive.

The Evidence

It is a commonly held myth that at a certain age, perhaps at 65 years, a person's sexual activity diminishes and older people become neither sexually capable nor sexually arousable. As the subject of sexual activity slowly becomes less of a taboo subject more evidence becomes available of older people's sexual experiences. Physiologically the woman's sex drive is not necessarily affected by the menopause and, despite the cessation of ovulation, the libido is not always affected (Coni, Davison and Webster 1992). The physiology of normal ageing does mean that in men the arousal rate slows, the penis is less sensitive and the angle of erection lowers. In women the vulva and the vagina become less sensitive and may become drier. The number of orgasms achieved may also decrease, but a satisfying relationship is possible for most older people who wish to participate in sexual activity (Roberts 1989c).

Summing Up

Older people can continue to have an active and enjoyable sex life if they want one.

The Ageing Brain

The Allegation

All old people are 'forgetful' and find it difficult to learn anything new.

The Evidence

Many aspects of the ageing brain will be addressed in the psychology of ageing. It is important, though, to note the general physiological changes that take place. The normal ageing process does not include dementia, memory loss does not occur as a matter of course and intelligence is not affected by age. The few changes in the brain noted at post mortem include weight loss, enlarged ventricles, thickening of the blood vessels and meninges and reduced numbers of neurotransmitters. These changes result in forgetfulness, a lengthening in reaction time, and an ability to learn but at a slower pace (Roberts 1989d).

Summing Up

Older people can learn new things but are slower and take longer to absorb the information.

Balance

The Allegation

Older people fall frequently because they are unstable on their feet.

The Evidence

Admissions of older people to Accident and Emergency departments are frequently due to falls. It is accepted almost as part of the ageing process and this indeed can be confirmed statistically; 20 per cent of older men and 40 per cent of older women will have fallen for a variety of reasons (Roberts 1989d). Nearly half of these are caused by environmental factors such as uneven pavements, rucked-up carpets or trailing flexes (Roberts 1989d). Some people are affected as the mechanics of balance and postural control deteriorate; the remaining bulk of incidents are caused either because of multiple pathology or active illness; this includes transient ischaemic attack and cardiac problems.

Summing Up

Older people do fall more than younger people and it is often due to instability, which is a natural progression of old age.

The Endocrine System

The Allegation

The hormone system remains the same throughout life, except when women go through 'the change'.

The Evidence

Different parts of the endocrine system appear to respond to the ageing process differently. The pituitary, which regulates all other endocrine organs, appears to maintain its functions throughout the person's life span (Bromley 1988). The thyroid, however, does atrophy with age. A reduction in its functioning means that the regulating of body energy and metabolism changes (Roberts 1990). This increases the chances of an older person suffering from myxoedema with confusion resulting in a low body temperature (Bromley 1988). It is well known and acknowledged that the gonads in women have degenerative changes at around the age of 50, this bringing about the cessation of the menstrual cycle and the ability to bear children. Degeneration of the male hormones is not so dramatic but does occur with age. Although a man in his 80s will produce viable sperm they will be fewer in quantity.

Summing Up

Hormonal changes occur which can affect how the whole body works.

THE VISUAL EFFECT OF AGEING

The most obvious sign of ageing is the older person's outward appearance. For the media and cosmetic companies the ageing process commences at about 18 years old. Creams to moisten, dewrinkle, turn grey hair dark and even make hair grow are sold in Western society, being bought with great enthusiasm in the hope that they will delay or reverse the signs of ageing.

In spite of the multimillion pound trade in these products few have ever been proved to have a permanent effect. Wrinkles will occur with the loss of subcutaneous fat and overexposure to sunlight. Grey hair is also considered a telltale sign of ageing yet this, along with balding in men, can occur at a very young age. Conversely, hair growth increases on certain parts of the body, notably ears, nostrils and eyebrows in men, chin, upper lip and around the nipples in women (Roberts 1986). The physical appearance of older people does affect how they are perceived and care professionals should be aware of this.

NORMAL PSYCHOLOGY IN THE OLDER PERSON

Identifying psychological changes due to the ageing process has caused researchers some concern in recent years; separating out and identifying those changes that are due purely to age and not life events is a very difficult process. There are two main methods of data collection. First, longitudinal studies have been used for nearly 80 years; in these studies the same cohort is studied repeatedly over a number of years. A well known example of this was the ITV documentary series '7 Plus', which was first filmed in the 1960s. This featured a number of children from different social backgrounds who were revisited every 7 years. Secondly, cross-sectional studies are used to analyse the psychology of ageing. These are conducted with a single cohort of people of different ages, with the study being conducted at one time giving a 'snapshot' measurement.

COGNITIVE ABILITY

There are enormous differences in the life experience of young children today, compared to that experienced by people who are now 'old'. They were children either in the First World War or during the great depression of the 1930s and will have been exposed to very different life experiences. In particular they will have had a different kind of education. The unknowledgeable person may assume from this that older people today are not so intelligent as younger people, but this is not so. The Intelligence Quotient (IQ) is the ratio of mental age to chronological age multiplied by 100. This method of measuring a person's intelligence shows that their IQ continues to develop until they reach school age and then it remains fairly stable, but it can increase even in later life if they are motivated to achieve (Hilgard, Atkinson and Atkinson 1979). There are differences, however, in what the older person is able to achieve with a marked deterioration in the older person's ability to do things that require quickness of response in perception or word fluency. Specific abilities relating to general knowledge show little change and, if a person has been in a particularly intellectually demanding job, their mental ability appears to remain unchanged. The effect of physical pathology, especially strokes or other disorders of the brain, will cause a decrease in the person's intellectual ability; yet ability can be helped to be preserved and improved or maintained in all older people if they are intellectually stimulated (Hilgard et al 1979).

MEMORY

When working solely with people who have dementia it is easy to slip into the belief that losing one's memory is a natural part of the ageing process. It is acknowledged that the cells of the cerebral cortex do not replace themselves as do other cells in the body, but there is little loss of primary memory in normal ageing. However, there is a fall in the ability to encode information from long-term memory, compounded by physical deterioration in visual, auditory or tactile stimulation. Learning new, unfamiliar material may cause problems as this is intertwined with the cognitive ability to learn new abstract things. The older person's ability to absorb and process complex new information and integrate it into their mind causes the difficulties associated with 'normal' old age; this contrasts with the durability of material that has been 'overlearned' and stays within the memory. It is this distinction that accounts for the difference between the efficiency of long-term and short-term memory. Therefore, being able to sing songs learned during childhood will remain with the person longer than the words of a song heard on the radio within the previous week. This is not due to dementia but the normal ageing process (Hartley, Harker and Walsh 1980). It is also important to acknowledge that familiarity with the material will affect how older people deal with it; old-fashioned words are more familiar to older people than new words, which are not so easily remembered (Barrett and Wright 1981). Care professionals need to be aware of the number of modern jargon words (e.g. loo/toilet, stereo/record player, video/film) that they use in daily conversation and make an effort to use language that is appropriate to their clients.

AGE AND PERSONALITY

The work of identifying personality types has become fundamental to the study of psychology. Two of the most famous theories of personality are Sigmund Freud's 'Psychoanalytic Theory' and Carl Rogers' 'Self Actualisation Theory' (Hilgard et al 1977). Theories about the formation of personality do not necessarily help to explain the effect of ageing on personality. The most frequently noticed change is a greater introversion as the person becomes older. Other traits, such as thoughtfulness and tolerance, show positive changes, and an older person's self-confidence and openness appear to remain unchanged (Choun, Nicholson and Foss 1983). This evidence may surprise some carers, given that popular belief states that older people lose their self-confidence. It seems from many longitudinal studies that very little of the person's personality is affected by age, but that life events breed certain attitudes and approaches. It could therefore be speculated that the introversion of the current generation of older people, particularly women, might change in future as career-minded women retire and become older (Choun et al 1983).

There is a stereotype of the satisfaction with life felt by older people; they are frequently viewed as 'grumpy, miserable and hard to please'. A variety of studies in a number of different towns and counties continue to show that the normal ageing process does not affect the satisfaction of an older person with their lifestyle. Older people are generally quite satisfied with their lifestyle in relation to the satisfaction levels of younger people (Choun et al 1983) but are less able to cope with unexpected events and crises.

THE PROCESS OF DYING

Older people are more frequently faced with the event of death than younger people. As years pass and friends and relatives die the older person must often contemplate their own mortality; or do they? Death is approached in many different ways; some people simply accept it in a matter-of-fact way, some become angry, some depressed and some do not accept the inevitability of death at all. The person's attitude to death will depend on their premorbid personality, and their preparation for dying will depend on this. It is recognised that people prepare for the terminal stages of their life and, even without being told directly, often have a sense of the impending event. Older people often find that they have no one to discuss death with and that the expression of their fears and anxieties is inhibited (Scrutton 1989). People are often ritualistic about preparing themselves for death, and it is within the limits of normal ageing for the person to hand over responsibilities to others, make arrangements for others and put 'their house in order'. This tends to give the person a feeling of control and completeness, allowing them to enter the terminal stage of life at peace with the world.

SOCIAL ASPECTS OF AGEING

The Older Person in the Family

What is old? Who is old? When does someone become old? In everyday life the answers to these questions are often based around the ability to claim the State Retirement Pension. At the magical age of 65 years a man can change from being a useful member of a company or workforce and become an 'old age pensioner', irrespective of his mental agility or physical fitness. A negative stereotype is attached to old age in this society and is in marked contrast to the status accorded to older people in other cultures (Patrick and Scambler 1984).

Family relationships have altered over the past 50 years in the United Kingdom, improved life expectancy and smaller families have altered the traditional family and the matriarchal role of the elderly grandmother figure is rarely found. The extended family now includes more neighbours and 'non-relatives' as people migrate all over the country with their work (Bromley 1988). Although some families may continue in the traditional style, with grandmother helping to care for the young family, many grandmothers are themselves working full-time until retirement, and so traditional support mechanisms are eroded.

Many older people live alone. In 1978 40 per cent of people over 70 years of age were living alone and considered to be isolated. The term 'isolated', however, does not describe lifestyle and is in itself a term that needs defining. One study suggested that to be isolated would include people who had taken part in less than 20 10-minute conversations during the previous week. Using this definition 60 per cent of older people are isolated (Tunstall 1966). This definition could apply just as easily to people living in their own homes or to people who live in institutions; administering physical care on a routine basis often does not include sitting down and chatting to the person. Like a railway station, a residential care setting can be a very busy, but a very lonely place.

Growing Old and the Class Structure

In Victorian England differences in the health and life expectancy of people from different social classes was quite distinct. The Victorians were very familiar with the vicious circle of poverty causing disease and disease causing poverty. However, this was all changed in 1948 when the National Health Service was created and health care became free to all. In spite of this there are still differences in how many people reach old age from different social classes. These differences relate to the factors that influence their health care status throughout adult life. Evidence shows that predisposing factors associated with the major diseases, such as heart disease, are found to be more common in Social Classes IV and V. These factors include poor diet, stress, smoking, atmospheric pollution and housing. A lack of knowledge about keeping healthy also compounds these factors, making disease and death at a younger age more likely among the 'working classes' (Patrick and Scambler 1984).

Women are more likely to live longer than men, regardless of their social class, with approximately 64 elderly men to every 100 elderly women (Bromley 1988). The sex differentials widen with increasing age, women constituting 80 per cent of the over-85 age group. The very frail elderly group in any setting will therefore be predominantly women.

Ageism – the New Discrimination

Contrary to popular belief, British society has never had a high opinion of the old: they have never been cossetted or venerated as in some cultures. They have always been depicted as a burden to society and have never had a voice in decision-making settings. They are often thought of as nonproductive members of society and less worthy of care than other groups. This is demonstrated quite clearly in many health and social care services, where the care of older people is perceived by managers and policy makers as an area where the quality and quantity of the staff may not need to be the same as in units of critical care or child protection. Ageism is rife in society for both the 'young old' and the 'very old'. Problems begin before retirement; the rate of redundancy for men over 40 years is twice that for men under 40 years (Carver and Liddiard 1982). Managers hold beliefs that older employees are forgetful, inflexible or expensive. The government does not produce statistics on age-related appointments or redundancies and so much of the opinion is unsupported (Patrick and Scambler 1984). Eligibility for some benefits stops at the age of 65 years as the person will then receive a retirement pension; this is regardless of the fact that their circumstances may not have changed.

Positive Ageing – A Possible Option

Many older people live in an institutional setting, but far more remain in their own homes. Some of these will have a disability of some description and yet they cope well and do not anticipate any other option. Statistics seem to highlight negative attitudes; for example, research shows that of 1121 people aged over 75 years in East Anglia, 35 per cent were unable to cook their main meal, 36 per cent were unable to shop and 13 per cent were incontinent of urine. These figures paint a rather depressing picture of the lifestyle of older people in East Anglia (Coni, Davison and Webster 1992) and perhaps confirm the fears and anxieties of people who are in their late 60s that, within 10 years, they have a one in three chance of being unable to get out of the house or cook and could also be incontinent. Statistics can be reframed to show another picture of future prospects for people who are looking towards old age: 65 per cent of people who are aged 75 years or over will still be able to cook their own meals, 64 per cent of people will still be going out of the house and shopping and 87 per cent will still be continent.

HEALTH PROMOTION

Health promotion has come to the forefront of health care in the 1990s, but it is rarely associated with the care of people with dementia. The document, *The Health of the Nation* (DOH 1991), highlights five areas of health care in England that should be addressed by health care professionals.

1. Coronary heart disease and stroke
2. Cancers
3. Mental illness
4. Accidents
5. HIV/Aids and sexual health

It is the government's intention that the incidence of these health issues should be reduced by the year 2000. All the other parts of the United Kingdom have similar documents that highlight the health care issues for them. Although all the general categories can include older people, there is only one target that could be directly linked to people with dementia. The first mental illness target is:

> Improve significantly the health, social functioning and quality of life of people who are mentally ill.

Health promotion for people with dementia should, therefore, include strategies to ensure that their quality of life is maintained in whatever way is appropriate and the global topic of health promotion should become specific in its interpretation, considering health promotion issues which relate to people who have dementia. The final part of this chapter will look at ways in which health promotion targets can be interpreted in the care of someone with dementia.

KEEPING ACTIVE AND MOBILE

Although it has already been acknowledged that there are changes in connective tissue as one ages, including the slowing of collagen synthesis and the decrease in elastic tissue, with a consequence of stiffer tendons, there are also sociological changes that affect mobility. Domestic life in the 1990s is not as physically arduous as it was in the 1920s. Hand washing, using a mangle, beating the carpets, walking everywhere and pushing bulky prams have all been replaced by highly sophisticated mechanical and electrical substitutes, giving people who work at home more 'leisure' time and less need to be involved in physical 'work'. As a person ages, the problem is likely to be compounded. When older people complain that they no longer have the energy they used to have it is rarely a physiological consequence of ageing, but is due to a decline in activity. This decline can be slowed and largely prevented by continuing physical exercise (Roberts 1988b). The type of exercise to be encouraged should be gentle, with walking being an ideal example. It can usually be fitted in to normal daily life and, if the person is able to move independently, they should be able to start at their own pace and build up to a walk of about 20 minutes twice a day (Roberts 1988b). Swimming is also good exercise, as it improves suppleness of joints and strengthens stamina. Cycling is a hobby enjoyed by many and if people have taken part in the past they may enjoy it again. There are many popular fitness activities which are followed by many young people, such as aerobics, step and Callanetics™. Older people wanting to join these activities should ensure that they are fit enough to participate, as they can be very demanding and sometimes damaging to the musculoskeletal system. An exercise course that has been designed especially for older people and disabled people is 'Extend'; classes are run nationally by qualified instructors who work to exercise schedules that avoid jerky movement or aerobic activity and are paced to suit the participants. It is vital that the level of activity is appropriate to the level of ability of the group, and that they are not made to feel self-conscious. The physiotherapy service would be the most appropriate profession to contact for advice and guidance about the introduction of activities, either at home or within an institution.

Keeping Flexible

As an older person's physical and mental health deteriorates there are increasing reasons to ensure they are kept as active as possible, for as long as possible. If limbs are not used, due to a cerebral vascular accident, arthritis or perhaps due to advancing dementia, the muscles may go into spasm and contractures may occur. They will continue to debilitate the older person unless active preventative measures are taken; these measures may include passive movement of the limbs, active movement if the person is able to follow instructions, and drugs to alleviate the pains and the spasm. The community nursing and physiotherapy services would be able to advise on the care for individual people with this problem. If it can be prevented and the person is able to remain ambulant, it will not only ensure a more independent and pain-free life for them, it will reduce the level of care required to be given and prevent complications from immobility, which could include pressure sores, chest infections, inability to feed and urinary tract infections. The person who has some mobility can ensure that they protect their flexibility by being encouraged to do more for themselves, perhaps to go with the home care professional to the shops, even though it may be slower and there is no obvious intellectual advantage. Within a residential setting people might be encouraged to collect their own food, help push the tea trolley or walk to the toilet with assistance rather than taking the 'quicker' wheelchair. These activities may present as time consuming but the time saved in the future might be immeasurable.

Continence

As the evidence within the chapter has already identified, incontinence is not a consequence of the ageing process, but 10–13 per cent of older people do have an incontinence problem and many of these will also have dementia. Many older people are embarrassed about their incontinence, having a misapprehension that it is an untreatable consequence of old age (WHO 1989). This is not correct. Anyone who suffers from incontinence, wherever they live or whatever other diseases they have, should receive appropriate assessment and treatment or equipment. In the United Kingdom a Continence Advisory Service has been taking the lead by offering specialist advice for the past 10 years (Roe 1993). It should not be accepted that putting a pad on someone is continence management; this is nothing more than incontinence control. The causes of incontinence, including stress, an atonic bladder, urgency, overflow and functional dysfunction, need accurate diagnosis and appropriate intervention. These interventions may include pelvic floor exercises and bladder training, e.g. a bladder voidance routine, which is not the same as the ritualistic 'toiletting routine' seen in some residential units. This bladder training is designed around an individual and depends on their baseline assessment, observation and the identification of trigger behaviour. It will take account of the person's orientation to the environment, medication and fluid intake. If the problem cannot be rectified, which in dementia may be inevitable, a variety of appliances should be considered with the advice of the continence advisory service. Intermittent or indwelling catheterisation may be necessary but only as a last resort. Promoting continence is a valuable and positive intervention for all older people and the

Continence Advisory Service should be contacted and their advice sought in all continence problems. It should not be a presumption that nothing can be done.

The Risk of Pressure Sores

A decubitus ulcer or pressure sore is tissue necrosis caused by occlusion of the local blood supply, and can occur on any bony prominence (Birchall 1993). A number of factors increase the risk of a person developing a sore and it is important to ensure that these factors are identified and positive health promotion procedures introduced to prevent older people suffering unnecessarily. A person does not have to be bed-bound to be at risk from developing pressure sores; exacerbating factors include both intrinsic and extrinsic factors, as follows.

- Immobility due to paralysis, arthritis, contraction, pain, bed rest or sedation.
- Altered consciousness.
- Loss of sensation, e.g. hemiparesis, peripheral neuropathy.
- Thinning dermis – due to poor circulation, steroid therapy.
- Debilitating disorders.
- Malnutrition – due to dietary deficiency.
- Dehydration.
- Incontinence.
- Being over 70 years of age.

- Poor lifting – dragging of people causing friction.
- Lack of exercise and mobility.
- Hard beds and chairs.
- Hard, over-dry underwear or sheets.
- Incontinence pads not being changed.

A qualified nurse, using a recognised pressure sore risk assessment tool such as the Waterlow Risk Assessment, the Pressure Sore Prediction Score or the Norton Scale (Birchall 1993) can identify the likelihood of pressure sores occurring. The appropriate care can then be implemented depending on the severity of the problem, to prevent deterioration of the skin. The care of any older person who is frail should always include the following.

- Good nutrition and hydration.
- Good skin cleansing techniques avoiding rubbing delicate skin.
- Prompt changing of soiled clothing.

- Appropriate pain control to prevent immobility.
- Regular position change both in bed and in the chair – every 2 hours.
- Appropriate bed and chair pressure relieving equipment, e.g. Propads, Spenco pads, Pegasus, etc. (Malone 1992).
- Minimising the use of wheelchairs as permanent seating.

Wherever there are older people who are at risk, health promotion should include pressure area risk assessment. Community nursing services would be the specialist advisers most appropriately placed to support Social Services department staff, who work with people either in their own homes or in residential settings, where there is no direct access to qualified nursing staff.

Nutrition

It is commonly supposed that the Western World suffers little mal-nutrition; that this is the province of the developing countries. Such a statement is inaccurate: older people in the United Kingdom do suffer malnutrition for a variety of reasons. In a recent survey by the King's Fund Centre more than 44 per cent of medical patients are malnourished on admission to hospital and prolonged hospital stay can cause malnutrition to develop for the first time (Lennard-Jones 1992). It is important to be aware of the nutritional needs of the older person when managing a service for a client group where the ability to eat a normal diet may be impaired. The Department of Health released a report of dietary values in 1991 to provide guidance on appropriate dietary com-position, and yet these guidelines have been condemned as being inappropriate to meet the needs of the older person (Wynne and Wynne 1993). Dietary supplements are available both from the pharmacist and on prescription if the person is not able to eat a normal diet, but where an older person has the ability to masticate, a 'normal' diet should be encouraged. Older people living at home should favour a diet that includes the basic requirements of protein, carbohydrates, fats and vitamins. If the person is able, they should be encouraged to remain in control of their own diet and food preparation as a way of main-taining their interest in cooking and keeping their fingers nimble. However, if there is only one person living on their own it may be more practical to purchase readymade meals: where this is the case it is important to ensure that these will provide an adequate nutritional intake. Information on the dietary requirements of older people can be obtained through the Health Authority Dietitian Service. Some basic information and menu ideas may also be available from the Health

Promotion department. Where care professionals are involved with people from an ethnic minority it is important that their dietary preferences are respected, that any rules relating to food and food preparation are honoured while still ensuring a wholesome diet.

It is important for the older person to remain nutritionally complete. It helps fight infections, disease and pressure sores and promotes activity. For the care professional it must be a cost-effective strategy to keep people well nourished in order to maintain their independence.

ACTION FOR CHANGE

1. Using the material in this chapter as a basis, compile a list of questions on 'normal ageing' to use as a basis for discussion at a staff meeting.
2. Conduct an audit within your service that looks at the number of conversations a sample of clients have each day – with each other and with the staff. Discuss your findings within the staff group; are any of the clients socially isolated?
3. Listen to the language and terminology used by your colleagues within your place of work. Is it in keeping with the generation of your client group? Make a list of the words you come across in a week that older people may not easily recognise. Decide if the use of these words is essential for the efficient running of the service; if not, try to discourage their use.
4. Review the laxative regime of clients; discuss with them, the medical staff and dietitians if there are any opportunities available to reduce their use.
5. Discuss in the staff team the attitudes towards appearance and age. Play a social game of guessing people's ages. Make positive statements about their appearance in respect of the ageing process.
6. Review the physical activity of an older person within your service. How much physical activity do they do? Can it be improved upon by changing routines, or through the way staff care for them?
7. Look through the accident report book. How many falls have there been in the past month and what action was taken? Could anything be done to minimise the number of falls? Are there any restrictions in the unit to prevent falls, which also impinge on the older person's civil liberty? Can you justify them?
8. Review the way that you assess the risk of pressure sores, look at the options of pressure area assessment tools and with appropriately qualified nursing staff decide on which best suits the needs of the unit. Decide on an action plan to implement the assessment procedure. If

you already assess clients regularly, review the effectiveness of the tool by looking at whether the number of pressure sores has decreased over the past few months.

REFERENCES

Barrett T R and Wright H (1981) Age related facilitation in recall following semantic processing. *Journal of Gerontology* **36**: 194–99.

Birchall L (1993) Making sense of pressure sore prediction calculators. *Nursing Times* **89**(18): 34–37.

British National Formulary (1993) *British National Formulary*, Number 25. London: British Medical Association.

Bromley D B (1988) *Human Ageing. An Introduction to Gerontology*. London: Pelican.

Carver V and Liddiard P (1982) *An Ageing Population*. Kent: Open University.

Choun S H, Nicolson J and Foss B. (eds) (1983) Age differences and age changes. *Psychology Survey No. 4*. London: British Psychological Society.

Coni N, Davison W and Webster S (1992) *Ageing: the Facts* Oxford: Oxford University Press.

Department of Health (1991) *The Health of the Nation*. London: HMSO.

Ebersole P and Hess P (1985) *Towards Healthy Ageing: Human Needs and Nursing Response*, 2nd edn. Toronto: Mosby.

Hartley J T, Harker J O and Walsh D A (1980) Contemporary issues and new directions in adult development of learning and memory. In: Poon L W (ed.) *Ageing in the 1980s*. Washington: American Psychological Association.

Hilgard E, Atkinson R and Atkinson R (1979) *Introduction to Psychology*, 7th edn. New York: Harcourt Brace Jovanovich

Hofman A, Roca W and Brayne C (1991) The prevalence of dementia in Europe: A collaborative study. *International Journal of Epidemiology* **20**: 736–45.

Lennard-Jones J E (1992) *A Positive Approach to Nutrition as a Treatment*. London: King's Fund Centre.

Malone C (1992) Intensive pressures. *Nursing Times* **88**(36): 57–62.

McMahon R (1992) *Nursing at Night*. London: Scutari Press.

Norman L (1989) *The Reflexology Handbook*. Bath: Piakus.

Patrick D and Scambler G (1984) *Sociology as Applied to Medicine*. Eastbourne: Baillière Tindall.

Roberts A (1986) Senior systems of life no. 1. *Nursing Times* **82**(16): 39–42.

Roberts A (1987) Senior systems of life no. 10. *Nursing Times* **83**(2): 35–38.

Roberts A (1988a) Senior systems of life no. 24. *Nursing Times* **84**(14): 43–45.

Roberts A (1988b) Senior systems of life no. 30. *Nursing Times* **84**(45): 65–68.

Roberts A (1989a) Senior systems of life no. 32. *Nursing Times* **85**(2): 45–48.

Roberts A (1989b) Senior systems of life no. 34. *Nursing Times* **85**(10).

Roberts A (1989c) Senior systems of life no. 37. *Nursing Times* **85**(24): 65–68.

Roberts A (1989d) Senior systems of life no. 43. *Nursing Times* **85**(49): 57–60.

Roberts A (1990) Senior systems of life no. 50. *Nursing Times* **86**(28): 63–66.

Roe B (1993) Promoting continence in Denmark and the UK. *Nursing Standard* **7**(40): 28–30.

Scrutton S (1989) *Counselling Older People*. London: Edward Arnold.

Tunstall J (1966) *Old and Alone: A Sociological Study of Older People.* London: Routledge.

Van der Cammen T, Rai G and Exton-Smith A (1991) *Manual of Geriatric Medicine.* New York: Churchill Livingstone.

Warnes A M (1989) *Human Ageing and Later Life.* London: Edward Arnold.

World Health Organisation (1989) *Health of the Elderly. Technical Report 779.* Geneva: WHO.

Wynne A and Wynne M (1993) Catering concerns. *Nursing Times* **89**(20): 61–64.

3 The Environment
Its use as a therapeutic tool

The place were we live, no matter what our age or our mental state, affects how we feel about ourselves and how we relate to others. The environment of an institution also makes a statement about the value placed on the residents by the professionals in charge and by society. The design of buildings and the furnishings can set the tone for care and can contribute to or help to minimise difficult behaviour. Financial restraints will mean that it will always be necessary for staff to be able to substantiate requests for alterations or new furniture, by indicating how relevant these changes will be to the quality of life of the residents.

POINTS TO PONDER

- Remember the last time friends came to your home for a meal: the environment, the aura, the company; compare that experience to the last meal served in your care setting.

- Going shopping and parking the car in a multistorey car park is an everyday event. Think about an occasion when you could not remember which floor your car was on.

- Think about the last time you were in an unknown building and wanted to go to the toilet. How did you find your way?

- What types of music do your friends enjoy? How does it feel to be bombarded by a style that is not to your taste?

- Cast your mind back to your last visit to the dentist. Can you remember the atmosphere in the waiting room? Can you identify why it felt that way?

- What feelings do you experience when you enter a darkened room, which has shadows casting strange shapes on the floor?

- Do you find that tea tastes different in a china cup compared to a plastic beaker?

- How many photographs do you have at home of your family or special friends? What special things do you have on your bedside table?

WHAT MAKES A HOME?

We all have a different lifestyle; as individual as fingerprints. Our living rooms or bedroom space makes a statement about ourselves that will not be repeated. For many, the location of the house remains the same for most of the person's adult life; if a person is used to a large town, with the hustle and bustle of traffic, it would feel strange even for an able-bodied person to move to a rural area. The social cues of the familiar surroundings will enable a confused person to continue living in a manner that does not cause alarm, either to themselves or to others. It is only when the person is removed from their own environment and placed elsewhere that more problems appear. This will be relevant wherever the person is taken, either to a relative's home or to a residential setting. The services provided should therefore be relatively local, wherever possible (Kelly 1992).

On admission to care people are expected to mix and form relationships with people from widely different social backgrounds. It must be noted, therefore, that a person who is not confused could become very unsure of themselves if they were put into an environment that was not familiar to them either physically or socially.

It has been identified that there are two types of environment, the physical and the social, the former being a sum of those potentially changeable factors, and the latter referring to the potential communicating factors (Gravell 1988). Therefore a total environment which is satisfactory for one may not be for another, either because the physical or social factors or both are a mismatch. However, the art of professional care is to ensure that the environment as a whole, that has to cater for many different people, will meet the standards and expectations of the majority, thus allowing minor alterations to take place for people who have more unusual requirements.

The environment of a hospital has been identified by Wilson-Barnett (1976) to cause psychological stress to patients. The 'new' world, known to staff but not to patients, the new routine and perhaps a new language have all been acknowledged as a stress factor for people entering a general hospital. If it is accepted that old age may bring problems such as deteriorating eyesight, or a slowing of the learning process, then the effect of stress is magnified and the new level of anxiety may understandably be higher (Gravell 1988). When this is compounded by an inability to retain the new information at all, wandering, apparently aimlessly, can be the result (Stokes 1988a).

THE DESIGN OF THE HOME

For most care professionals there is rarely the opportunity to affect the design of their unit; for them it is literally laid down and cast in stone. However, it is important to acknowledge the effect of the design of a unit on confused people, regardless of where it is, or of which type (Fleming and Bowles 1987).

How the environment looks affects the atmosphere of the unit, although with very positive staff the most appalling conditions can be improved by the energy generated within the unit. If there is a general 'run down feeling' to the unit with poor decoration and inadequate maintenance, it can contribute to an air of neglect (Norman 1989). This in turn can affect the people who are having to live in the environment, by lowering their spirits and thus their self-esteem and their feeling of self-worth. This, in people who are able to articulate, may manifest in a presentation of mild depression. For people who cannot easily express themselves the manifestation of similar symptoms may be interpreted as a progression of the 'dementia'.

Ideally the size of the establishment should be for no more than 30 people in one unit, but if they are to be encouraged to remain independent the unit should be for no more than 10 (Wightman 1992). This maximises personal contact and minimises confusion by providing a more homely atmosphere and encouraging more personalised care.

The environment will also include the lounge or public domain. Traditionally, it has been expected that people living in a residential setting should accept that this would include a large amount of time being spent in the company of others, many of whom they will not know. Studies have identified, however, that older people who are able to offer an opinion stated that they preferred, on the whole, to lead a more private life (Brearly 1990). There is no reason to believe that older people who cannot communicate their preference to care professionals have a different perspective. Therefore, any residential setting or family home, for an older person, should allow for a balance of 'public' and private space.

FURNISHINGS AND ACCESSORIES

The type of large furniture chosen for a residential setting for people with a dementing type of illness will not only affect their physical comfort, but can alter the behaviour they exhibit (Fleming and Bowles 1987). The choice of armchairs usually revolves around whether the chair should be covered with a fabric or a plastic coated material. It is easy to think automatically of incontinence problems as being the prime factor when making the decision within a unit, but if the philosophy is to manage continence in a proactive way, then the type of furniture covering used should not be an issue. The domesticity of furniture will assist in the overall objective to create a positive environment and will help to make people more relaxed, thus reducing antisocial behaviour (Coles 1992).

The style of large pieces of furniture must also be considered; care staff must be able to assist people out of chairs, yet the chairs must be comfortable (Oddy and Lodge 1993). Therefore, a variety should be available of different heights, shapes and sizes. Many people at home also have settees. These can be very popular, particularly if the person is ambulant (Phair and Good 1989), and they assist in improving conversation. The depth of the chair should be checked as even if the person is ambulant they might find difficulty in getting up if they only have short legs and the chair is deep! Some staff also hold the belief that people will not get up and wander if their feet do not touch the floor, thus, in their opinion, justifying the purchase of high 'geriatric chairs'. There is no research available to support this idea.

In many elderly care establishments around the country an invisible gremlin sets to work at night moving chairs against the walls or putting them into rows. Staff have also stated that residents like to see what is going on in the room and sitting against the wall enables this, or that it maximises the open space and so prevents tripping. Yet this seating design deters any kind of intercommunication, as people have to physically turn to speak to someone else. Most communication begins spontaneously following eye contact, and thus this disposition of furniture actively detracts from verbal stimulation. The most useful design is to have the chairs in groups of four (Sommer and Ross 1958). Chairs that have high wings should also be avoided, along with 'geriatric chairs', as they prevent eye contact (Gravell 1988). The position of the chairs should also allow passageways, for people who wish to move about (Kelly 1992).

Placing small tables in front of people when seated is also a practice often witnessed; this can cause agitation and stimulate the person to try to move it. If the person cannot quite understand the object in front of them it will cause them distress. The use of tables beside people is preferable; coffee tables are aesthetically more pleasing but can be the cause of falls if a person's vision is impaired, as they are below the line of sight.

Some older institutions have large day rooms, where room dividers or Welsh dressers can enhance the homely environment and can also be used as bookshelves or cutlery stores (Marston and Gupta 1977; Phair and Good 1989). If the space is large this can add to confusion as people cannot identify themselves with the unit; thus wandering can occur, as people try to find out where they are (Stokes 1988a).

The type of bed supplied in an institutional setting is usually either a single divan or a full nursing bed with backrest and metal frame. Both types are, possibly, quite alien to older people who may have been married for many years and shared a double bed. People who are confused may not be able to identify the unfamiliar feeling of a hard institutional bed, so may become anxious and more confused and nocturnal disturbance may result (Stokes 1988a). Conversely, a mattress only has a life of about 7 years and if beds are also old and sagging this will interfere with the sleep pattern. In a continuing care setting where space allows, and where there is no clinical reason for a hospital style bed, it may help the person feel more settled if they not only have their own wardrobe, but also their own comfortable double bed.

The accompanying furniture in the bedroom should be serviceable but homely. There is no logical reason why people who are in bed spaces, or ideally their own rooms, still need a hospital bedside locker! They are confusing and awkward for the most able-bodied people and, as they are usually on wheels, can easily change location if a person is prone to furniture removals. A wardrobe, perhaps secured to the wall for safety, a chest of drawers and a bedside cabinet are familiar pieces of furniture in most homes. At least one item should also have a lockable drawer for the person's private effects that are 'precious' to them. A mirror should also be standard equipment to ensure that the person can reorientate themselves to who they are, whenever they feel the need.

Walking along corridors or circular routes created by open doors will effectively assist the 'wandering' person to be more settled. While wandering to the observer will often appear to be aimless, it is often purposeful to the participant (Stokes 1988a), but if people encounter locked doors they will become more agitated as they become more convinced that the thing they are seeking lies behind that particular locked door. Corridors must provide suitable stimulation, however, thus diverting the person's attention: perhaps a garden or large safe windows for them to view outside activity; but there must be chairs or places to encourage the person to rest as they might otherwise become exhausted (Norman 1987).

Within the care setting harsh rooms can be softened with pictures, ornaments or pieces of incidental furniture. These should be in keeping with the generation of the residents. Modern abstract paintings may stimulate discussion for the person who is cognitively alert; however, for those who have difficulty with interpretation of normal visual experiences, such pieces can be very disorientating and can, on occasions, be altered by the person's perception to become frightening.

SIGNPOSTING

Signposting is found to be useful for people who suffer with dementia, although for them to have most benefit its use should be accompanied by a training procedure. The signs are more successful if they are non-verbal and should be used appropriately. The appropriateness of the design of the sign to the age of the older person should also be considered. Symbols depicting male and female may not be easily identifiable; how-ever, literature about the design of information signs of 40 years ago is scanty (Kelly 1992). The particular colour is not relevant as long as it contrasts with the colour of the main door. Any signs used should be firmly fixed, as many people with dementia are tempted to remove these things (Calkins 1988). In isolation this is not a major problem, but the broader aspect of how the staff will react to the person who causes such damage should be the principal consideration.

There is also evidence that some units attempt to orientate people by painting lines on the floor to direct residents from main rooms to the toilet (Miller 1977). These lines, however, would have to be in bright colours as older people cannot distinguish pastel colours easily. This suggests that the ethos of the ward would become less domestic using such a method of orientation.

THE AROMA OF THE UNIT

Walking into a 'geriatric' ward of 10 or 15 years ago would automatically alert the nasal passages to the smell of urine and faeces, particularly first thing in the morning. Today continence aids and increased knowledge of care professionals should ensure that offensive smells are kept to a minimum. Of course, a smell in itself is unpleasant and if hygienic methods are not used bacteria can multiply very quickly. It is also not desirable for visitors and care staff, who have to go into the rooms and care for the person. However, at least for these two groups of people, exposure to unpleasant odour is intermittent. For the person living in the home or care setting, however, there is no respite. The knowledge that the sense of smell deteriorates with the advancement of a dementing illness (Rai et al 1989) should not distract the care professional from dealing with the problems of aroma effectively.

The smell of the unit will be noticed by visitors to the care setting. This can have a profound effect on how people perceive the standard of care, and in turn affect people's attitude towards the staff. If the feeling of 'poor care' is allowed to manifest, it will reflect in the relationships between care professionals and relatives and between the care professionals and other disciplines.

ACOUSTICS

The level of noise in an institutional setting is often high. A building where many people are working and living cannot exist without communication and movement, and thus noise. The use of radio, television or music decks is considered to be stimulating and indeed music therapy is becoming more popular, but stimulation of residents by the use of such media should be considered carefully. Imposing a certain type of music on a group of people can cause some to feel relaxed and at ease, and yet others to feel agitated and angry because the music is not to their taste (Bettiss 1993). Music was found by Bettiss to be very important to many people and was fundamental to their general well-being. These clients were able to articulate what types of music they enjoyed or to discuss pieces that brought back good or bad memories. People with dementia will identify pieces of music that they learned many years earlier and rhythm and rhyme will be recalled easily. However, the memories that they elicit may be positive or negative and care professionals have to be careful that people do not become distressed during the activity of singing. Songs commonly encouraged are those from the two World Wars. This should only be done if staff are aware of experiences that people have had, and then be skilled and competent enough to deal with the outcomes.

It should also be a fundamental philosphy of a unit that cares for older people that the radio is not put onto a channel for the staff's benefit, e.g. a pop station, or the televison is not on at the same time and is left to show children's cartoons causing a droning noise in the background. Loud noise can become troublesome even for the older person who is able-bodied, if they are expected to concentrate on more than one task (Hilgard, Atkinson and Atkinson 1979). Unexpected or unpredictable noise can affect people's ability to function even more than a constant loud noise and applying this to people with dementia, their ability to follow simple tasks could be improved if the correct atmosphere was created.

Ambient noise, or the general noise created by the living environment, may affect people with dementia in their ability to distinguish sounds and voices (Kelly 1992). Within a general hospital setting older people identified that the noise levels of the ward were among the items found to be most stressful both during the day and the night (Wilson-Barnett 1976; Davies and Peters 1983). This could be reflected within a care setting for older people with dementia as being significant. Conversely silence can lead to anxiety and tensions and, for some, the need to create noise (Stokes 1988b). If the unit is completely silent for long periods of time and there is no auditory stimulation, people may shout simply to create an atmosphere.

THE USE OF CARPETS

Floor covering can assist in dampening sounds and preventing echoes. The use of carpets is becoming more popular and they are now recognised as being an appropriate covering, particularly in the lounge (Handysides 1993). However, they are likely to become grossly contaminated and grow almost double the amount of micro-organisms than smooth floors (Kelly 1992). However, carpets are more comfortable, more pleasing to the eye and are slip resistant. This is important, as people mobilising with an altered gait can find polished floors difficult to walk on. The use of walking frames and wheelchairs can also be compromised with carpet, but if the pile is short the problems should almost be eliminated. Acoustic floor covering in the bedrooms ensures easy cleaning, while maintaining noise levels at a minimum (Phair and Good 1989), yet does not promote a domestic environment. With appropriate continence management and frequent cleaning, carpets should be present throughout the care setting and are now required in residential homes by the majority of registration units.

There are difficulties for some people with a dementing illness to differentiate between types of floor covering and being unable to judge depth, they may not be able to cross from one room to another, or they may try to 'step over' the edge of a carpet or squares or stripes on the floor, perceiving them as a change in level. To assist people to feel more confident in walking it might be more suitable to have fewer changes in floor

covering style. Some homes have adopted the principle that the sound of
the floor will assist in people recognising their own home environment,
therefore the halls have a different floor covering to the bedrooms
(Handysides 1993).

LIGHTING

The amount of lighting available in a care setting can affect quite
dramatically people's perception of their surroundings. Natural light is
obviously the most appropriate and large secure windows will enable
plenty of light and also an opportunity for people to watch the activities
outside. However, at night lighting can cast shadows, particularly in
bedrooms and, if a person has difficulty with perception, the fluctuation
of light casting shadows can cause illusions. This in turn can cause the
person to shout, telling the vision to leave the room (Stokes 1988b).
Alternatively the person may leave their room unable to explain what
they see (Stokes 1988b). Bedside lights are also sometimes difficult for
the person to switch on, and so compound the problems of shadows.
Fluorescent lighting is, traditionally, the type to be found in institutions.
Many of the older types cause glare, and overstimulate people. Modern
fluorescent lighting systems give enough 'candle power' to offer good
stable lighting. Older people who suffer from cataracts find that although
their vision is impaired the reception of light is enhanced and glare can
occur, either from natural or artificial light. They may shy away from
rooms, not because they are antisocial, but because they cannot cope with
brightness. Lighting should therefore be practical but not glaring and,
above all, should not cast shadows or encourage dark corners that
can be interpreted as images. Wall lighting, as a pleasant alternative,
can encourage a restful atmosphere, particularly in the evening (Phair and
Good 1989).

WALLCOVERING

Wallcovering and the colour of paint can also influence how people
conduct themselves in a care setting. Unfortunately, in most care settings
walls are painted magnolia. Wallpaper, particularly if it has large patterns,
can again cause difficulties for people with perceptual problems. One lady,
who was still living at home, kept seeing children coming out of the wall.
The community psychiatric nurse identified that the lady was misinter-
preting large flower-patterned wallpaper and was seeing the flowers as

figures. The local Rehabilitation Officer for the Visually Impaired may be able to give advice and thus help to ensure that these situations are minimised. Plain walls are arguably the most appropriate and pastel colours are least offensive to the vast majority of people. Also it has been recognised that people with a dementing illness may lose their ability to differentiate between colours, and so colour coding will only be successful if it is combined with other orientation cues (Calkins 1988). However, this can be used positively to disguise doors that should not be found easily by wandering people. Doors for cleaning cupboards, store rooms or sluices should be painted the same colour as the walls, and only doors that are significant, for instance, the toilet and bathroom, should be painted in a bright primary colour. Bedroom doors are probably more easily recognised by the person from personal identification objects, for example their name, a room number and a personal photograph on the door (Kelly 1992). To colour code too many different types of doors will only complicate the identification of rooms that are vital to be noted easily.

RESPECTING PRIVACY

Living in a domestic home, whether it is a flat, a bungalow or a bedsit, still gives the occupier the right to choose who they invite into their personal space and living area. Some people enjoy privacy more than others; for some being alone is depressing and isolating, for others it is energising and enables reflection. Older people have had a lifetime to understand themselves and learn what level of company they enjoy, and also what type of company they wish to have.

The problem of being admitted to a care setting is that people are forced to mix with others, whether they want to or not. The lack of privacy is identified by Davies and Peters (1983) as a significant reason for raised stress levels in an elderly care unit. Once again the subjects were cognitively intact and could understand what was happening around them. People who suffer from a dementing illness may not have the ability to understand what is happening and it is quite reasonable to suppose that this could cause an increased level of anxiety within older people. This is basic common sense, yet in many places 'Nightingale' wards are still used, with little or no effective partitioning to offer people their own space. Individual rooms are by far the most dignified way of caring for someone, as it gives them the opportunity to feel that they belong 'somewhere'. Staff also show people greater respect where there are single rooms, and promote privacy automatically (Norman 1987).

Offering physical care in the privacy of single rooms is made easier and unpleasant noises or aromas, that may affect others, can be kept private.

Raising a person's self-esteem and supporting their self-worth can be helped by ensuring that personal belongings are taken into the care setting with the older person. Familiarity helps to relieve anxiety and can assist in reality orientation. Marking the bedroom door with the person's own memorabilia may make it easier for them to find their bedroom; one gentleman had the emblem of his lifelong-supported football club put on the door (Hanley et al 1981).

To enable everyone to feel satisfied with the level of privacy may be difficult. Older people still regard privacy in an institution as a luxury and one that should not be expected; it is therefore not always addressed as an issue even by mentally able older people (Higgs, MacDonald and Ward 1992). Offering the person the opportunity to have their own key, even if they are labelled as 'severely confused', would be a test and offer a quantitative measure of the care professional's commitment to ensuring that the person can expect privacy. A drawer inside a cupboard within the room, which is lockable, can also allow the person the opportunity to retain some privacy.

Privacy also extends outside the bedroom. The number and style of bathrooms or toilets in a unit will encourage or destroy the opportunity for privacy. Ideally, each bedroom should have its own washbasin and, possibly, toilet. If people do have their own washing facilities it will also encourage better basic hygiene, whether conducted personally or by a care professional, as the facilities are to hand. The lack of privacy with toilet facilities can lead to older people finding it difficult to eliminate. Within the Western culture elimination activities are conducted in private and if someone is aware of people in another cubicle or on the other side of a door, they may withhold the act of excretion because of embarrassment, which can have serious consequences. If someone becomes constipated they can sometimes become more restless, as they continue to obtain and resist the desire to eliminate. If this continues abdominal distention, pain, loss of appetite, nausea and vomiting can occur and if the situation remains undetected the person can become dehydrated and thus more confused and agitated. Yet the person may still not be able to express to others the simple, yet fundamental, issue that has caused the problem.

There should be bedrooms which are large enough to take a double bed or two single beds if a person has a relationship which they wish to continue in the privacy of their own room.

MAINTAINING A PERSON'S IDENTITY

To maintain someone's personal identity, even if they are unable to do so themselves, is vital if individualised care is to be achieved. With respect to the environment, however, identity is shown by personal statements that are made by the people who are resident in a unit: by their furniture and the physical environment that is created around them. The number and types of artefacts and ornaments present in a continuing care setting will illustrate the staff's desire to see the unit as the resident's home. The obvious contribution to enabling people to feel at home is to encourage them to have their own bedroom furniture. This of course should extend, if clinically appropriate, to their own style and size of bed and their own bed linen. Many units are now using continental quilts, yet some older people find these quite alien. The resident's own furniture could also be used in the lounges of the unit; this is a particularly useful consideration if different noninstitutional furniture is desired but cannot be afforded by the unit. Most furniture can be treated to make it non-flammable; however, the use of furniture made of plastic foam should never be considered because of the toxic fumes generated (Wightman 1992). It must always be remembered why the need for familarity is important, and the relevance should be considered with relation to people wandering, apparently aimlessly, because they are trying to find their bearings (Stokes 1988b); this might manifest as increased anxiety, because they cannot piece information together, or as excessive shouting (Stokes 1988b).

Relatives and carers also need to feel that they can talk to their relatives in a private setting. To be able to discuss personal feelings only within the hearing of others is embarrassing and particularly inhibiting. A com-bination of available rooms, armchairs or bedrooms, or the chairs arranged in social circles, can help to solve this problem.

Personal and private space within an institutional environment is very difficult to achieve. However, if care professionals wish to promote privacy and the personal identity of the older people living there, ground rules such as knocking on the bedroom door each time staff enter, asking permission to interrupt if a question needs to be asked when people are talking and asking if the person objects when care is needed to be carried out, must be established. These fundamental rules convey respect for another person's privacy and personal identity and should be afforded to everyone, regardless of their clinical diagnosis.

TAKING RISKS

Life is full of risks. Everyone everywhere takes risks simply to stay alive. Staff risk their lives every day to get to the place where they are employed. However, care professionals are free and able to make decisions about the lifestyle that they lead and the consequent risks attached to it. People who suffer with a dementing illness are not free; they are trapped within a degenerating disease, and they are sometimes cared for in environments that take away their freedom to choose their own level of risk.

Statements about risk taking provoke thoughts and discussion about the legality, morality and ethical considerations surrounding the safety of patients with dementia, yet there are quite clearly three types of risk that can be identified when caring for older people.

1. The risk to the person because of the environment.
2. The risk to the person because of the degenerative nature of the illness affecting their own judgement within the environment.
3. The risk to the staff through offering care.

There are two elements within each of these three areas. The term 'risk' is used to mean that there is a chance, or possibility, or probability, that something might happen or that there is a chance something unpleasant or harmful may occur (Brearly 1990). Kelly (1992) states that one of the first considerations when designing a unit for people with dementia is safety and security; but there should also be a positive milieu. For some care professionals these two aspects may not blend happily. To consider the environment and risk under the three areas highlighted may enable these concepts to merge.

The risk to the person due to the degenerative nature of their disease will raise thoughts of wandering or leaving the gas on at home, but if the word 'risk' is changed to 'hazard' a more concrete or structural concept becomes evident. Hazards within a care setting may appear obvious: leaving water on the floor, not having a light bulb replaced thus leaving a dark corridor, leaving the bed brakes off or not reporting the frayed edge of the carpet; they are all relevant risks that are heightened because an older person with dementia, who may also have deteriorating eyesight, may not be able to accommodate. For example, an elderly man may have an altered gait due to Parkinson's disease, a cerebral vascular accident or advancing dementia, and so shuffle. This quite obviously would be hazardous if he was walking on the worn carpet and his foot became entangled. Practical or physical hazards are just as dangerous for older people with dementia as for anybody else; care professionals are accountable if deterioration in the fabric of an environment will put somebody at risk.

The person's mental state and capacity to function independently will affect their level of risk; risk areas usually concern 'wandering', or damaging oneself within a domestic area, e.g. with hot water in the bath or sharp knives. There are also risks involved in people's dressing ability. If, for example, an older person cannot tie their shoelaces they could fall and fracture their femur. The care professional has, therefore, a fundamental duty of care to promote safety from the most basic of aspects.

Caring environments can be designed to reduce risk in a constructive way. As has already been discussed, developing a safe pathway for people who wish to wander will ensure safety without endangering them. Having a garden within the unit will only enhance the pleasure of the walk without increasing the risk.

Restriction of a person will often cause an increase in their presenting behaviour, yet many methods are used because of the potential risk of the person's behaviour to themselves. The most common are baffle locks on the doors, coded locks or straightforward keys. Sadly, the use of armchairs that tip back and have lockable tables to prevent people getting up is still common in some institutions. The use of all these methods of restraint comes within the subject of the physical environment yet they are almost, if not wholly, unlawful and constitute false imprisonment unless justification in law can be shown (Dimond 1993). It is no more justifiable to keep someone locked in a chair because of the risk that they might fall than it is to lock someone in a house in case they are knocked down by a car (FOCUS 1992). The use of environmental restraints can also exacerbate the symptoms of their dementia and enforce helplessness, muscular atrophy, agitation and shouting (Stokes 1988b; FOCUS 1992). Suggestions as to how to control behaviour evident in dementia are contained throughout this book and strategies should be followed accordingly.

Ensuring that the environment is safe for care professionals is just as important, if people are to feel valued and if staff are not to experience long terms of sick leave because of damaged backs. The appropriate use of chairs has already been discussed, but there is evidence to suggest that care professionals expose themselves unnecessarily to damaging their backs. There are various methods by which the risk can be reduced, for example:

a. using two staff and not struggling to lift alone;
b. having appropriate lifting equipment;
c. assessing the resident's mobility individually;

d. not presuming dependence;
e. installing handrails in appropriate places and at appropriate heights, e.g. bathrooms, washrooms; and
f. ensuring that there are handrails in corridors (Oddy and Lodge 1993).

Bathrooms are an area within the care setting that provide an ideal measurement of risk against safety. The use of hoists or hydraulic baths will assist care professionals in reducing risks to their backs and will help in lifting and make the task of bathing a 'one-person job'. However, for people who have lost the ability to judge distance, have visual and perceptual degeneration and can only retain an instruction for 20 seconds, being elevated 6 feet in the air before being plunged into a bath of luke-warm water (because of the risk of scalding) can be very frightening. Staff must always be mindful that such routine activities using equipment to reduce the risk of injury can potentially increase anxiety and thus increase danger to the older person. At the same time staff should consider when using a hoist with a person who is physically independent but 'might get stuck in the bath', that to disarm and enforce dependency will only reinforce their feelings of poor self-worth and hopelessness.

TAKING RISKS IN A DOMESTIC SETTING

The physical environment, wherever it is, is a place full of risk. Yet the issue of risk is more complex than simply the physical manifestation of the unit. The real issue of risk is embroiled in the attitude of staff and how they perceive their role in 'protecting' or 'enabling' older people with dementia. Imagine for a moment an elderly lady who has a severe short-term memory deficit with a recall of about 20 seconds; she lives alone and lives on cat food, which is 'kindly' supplied by the neighbour. She also leaves the cooker on and buries any meals prepared for her in the garden. Do the care professionals put her into care as the risk to her own health is too great? Or do they 'mould' the environment of her home, i.e. disconnect the gas supply and supervise meals, etc. to enable her to stay at home, if this is where she wants to be? Within an institutional setting, do the staff lock the front door because 'they' might wander off and get lost; or are the doors left unlocked and any potential wanderers identified and appropriate management strategies adopted? The environment can assist in reducing the physical risk to older people with dementia but staff attitudes need to address the life risk issues.

A Home at Home

Since the implementation of the NHS and Community Care Act 1990, in 1993, the increasing emphasis is for people to be supported in their own homes for as long as possible. The number of nursing and residential beds, in theory, will decrease. For many, therefore, discussions about the effect of the environment on a person with dementia may seem super-fluous. This could not be further from the truth, as principles of good practice should be developed and moulded to suit every situation. Good practice can be transferred to a domestic setting whether it is a bungalow, a house or a flat. The fundamental difference is that the carer is not a professional person who has had years of training and support, but is often someone who has found themselves in a situation with the problem of understanding and coping with their change in lifestyle, their changing relationship with the person, loss and grief and an expectation by the Welfare State that they know how to manage a person with a dementing illness. Care professionals who have a conceptualised under-standing of cause and effect of behaviour can use their knowledge to advise, discuss and educate carers about the effects of the environment on the older person. The home is, of course, the carer's home too, and so discussion and suggestions about perhaps moving furniture or fencing in the garden would need to be approached with tact. In principle there are budgets available to adapt a home to meet disabled people's needs but finance is rationed, thus sometimes meaning a carer has to manage in a home that is not adapted to the standard of a home for a disabled person and without the appropriate aids. However, in many ways the mere fact of being at home can reduce the incidence of behavioural problems, simply because the person is in familiar surroundings and is aware, because of retention of concrete facts in their long-term memory of their environment. They already have their favourite armchair, and have their cup of tea at the time they want it and can reflect on orna-ments that have a personal meaning. External social cues also help to orientate the person, the time the postman calls, the mobile fish shop that always calls on a Wednesday and has done so for the past 10 years, and church bells ringing for 8 o'clock Mass on Sunday; all these factors help to orientate and enable the person to keep in touch. Nature itself acts as a social cue stimulus, with daffodils signifying Spring, or brown leaves identifying Autumn; and if the person has been in touch with the natural environment within his home this too can help in his orientation.

Many aspects of providing care within a home environment become extremely difficult, particularly because the carer is so emotionally involved and often physically exhausted. Alterations, gadgets, lifting aids, ramps, a continence service, all facilities enjoyed by the institution, can now be available to carers in their own homes under the provisions of the NHS and Community Care Act, provided that the need is identified (and the resources are available); but community staff should proactively assist in educating the carer, not reactively supporting when the situation gets out of control (Tothill 1992). It is vital that support continues, particularly when they are managing the situation to the best of their ability. If there is no more help obviously available when all measures have been implemented, the situation may continue to deteriorate and the carer may need to come to terms with the knowledge that residential care may become the only option (Phair 1991).

Creating a Positive Milieu

However sensitive or impervious someone is to a person's tone of voice, or the effect of the decoration of a room, few could deny that they have 'felt an atmosphere' when they have entered a meeting room, the doctor's waiting room or a friend's house when the occupants have just had a row. Older people who suffer from dementia are able to perceive atmosphere as able-bodied people, or indeed as babies, can and will respond accordingly. They may not be able to articulate their feelings but present them in other ways.

Because of their short-term memory deficits they will also have difficulty in forming relationships, yet once familiarity is established they often can continue, at a superficial level, to hold a conversation. To ensure that the atmosphere is positive and that people are encouraged to formulate social relationships, the environment in a care setting may need to be engineered. It has already been discussed how the layout of the furniture can encourage communication; inviting people to sit at the dining table in social groups of four is more natural than sitting alone or at large tables of eight. Mealtimes in some cultures are the hub of family life and allow for conversation and social stimulation, yet in the United Kingdom meals can be rushed. Within a care setting meals can be seen as no more than an opportunity to check that everybody is on the unit and ensure adequate dietary intake. Enhancing the social aspect of meals, by laying tables with mats, the correct cutlery, condiments and teapots, encouraging people to help themselves and each other will invite communication and social interaction. If a dispute erupts, this can be interpreted as a positive outcome as people are being enabled to express themselves as they might have done in the past (Brearly 1990). Promoting discussion about the meal enhances the person's autonomy and self-control, aids communication and promotes independence (Phair and Good 1989). Even when people are severely disabled they can be brought to the table and transferred to a dining room chair, offered a cloth napkin and, if appropriate, fed at their own pace by a care professional who sits next to them and gives the non-verbal positive messages that the meal is the person's time, and not a task for staff. Some people have difficulty with mastication and a soft diet may be necessary, but this action reduces the need to chew and so could paradoxically compound the problem. Because of this liquidised food should be avoided, if at all possible.

The social interaction of the care setting can be enhanced by the provision of clocks that can be seen easily and that tell the correct time, also by the provision of daily newspapers that people are encouraged to look at.

Reality orientation boards have become a popular feature in residential settings for people who suffer with dementia, giving details of the date, weather and where the unit is (Holden and Woods 1982), yet there are some who dispute their validity and value, as the weather can be seen from the window, an address can often mean nothing and can able-bodied people remember the date anyway (Kelly 1992)? The boards also create an institutional 'air' simply by their imposing nature on the wall of the lounge.

Creating an environment that limits the distress it causes to people who are confused and unable to synthesise a great deal of new information is often hampered by external forces, money and lack of will power being two main factors. However, as it is acknowledged that the ability of the person to redefine their behaviour to suit the setting is very limited, the appropriate avenue to ensure that the needs and desires of the people are met must be towards manipulating the environment to suit the older person (Miller 1977). In the end, the provision of an environment that is appropriately designed and ergonomically correct will not only assist the older person, but will assist staff in the ability to offer appropriate specialised care for people with dementia.

The areas discussed and avenues highlighted are superficially simple, but until the implications of changes to the environment can be expressed to managers and financiers from a knowledge-based perspective, it may be difficult to initiate change. Many alterations can be made easily with the existing context of the unit and staff establishment. Creating an environment that is positive and homely is a clear statement to the world about the value that care professionals place on the people in their care. This may take years to achieve but can be done if it is desired by the care professional.

ACTION FOR CHANGE

1. Review the accident book and consider how many incidents are due to the environment.

2. Within continuing care settings consider how many personal possessions the residents have. Who has none? Why is that? What personal possessions could short-stay or respite care people be encouraged to bring in to the unit?

3. What pieces of furniture are domestic in nature? Why are some items not domestic? What would you not have in your own home – why?

4. If a resident regularly gets up and wanders at night, go and sit in their room; see where the shadows are, what noises can be heard and what things cannot easily be understood.

5. Encourage a member of staff to put on a pair of glasses that have been smeared in vaseline. How 'user friendly' is the environment if you cannot see exactly where everything is?

6. Ask someone who does not know the unit to try to find specific rooms, e.g. the toilet or the office, using the signposts. Evaluate their effectiveness.

7. If the unit is locked or if any rooms (other than cleaning cupboards) are locked, sit and observe for 2 hours. How many people try to leave or enter the rooms? Reflect on your findings and discuss alternative management strategies accordingly.

REFERENCES

Bettiss C (1993) Caution: Music at work. *Elderly Care* 5(1): 20–22.

Brearly C (1990) *Working in Residential Homes for Older People*. London: Routledge.

Calkins M P (1988) *Design for Dementia*. Maryland: National Health Publishing.

Coles (1992) The Nature of Dementia with some Implications for Design. In: Coles R et al. (1992) *Signposts not Barriers*. Stirling: University of Stirling Dementia Services Development Centre.

Davies A and Peters M (1983) Stresses of hospitalization in the elderly: nurses' and patients' perceptions. *Journal of Advanced Nursing* 8: 99–105.

Dimond B (1993) A case of false imprisonment. *Elderly Care* 5(1): 18–19.

Fleming R W and Bowles J R (1987) Units for the confused and disturbed elderly: development, design, programming and evaluation. *Australian Journal on Aging* 6(4): 125–32.

FOCUS RCN (1992) *Focus on Restraint*, 2nd edn. London: Royal College of Nursing.

Gravell R (1988) *Communication Problems in Elderly People* Beckenham: Croom Helm.

Handysides S (1993) Helping people with dementia feel at home. *British Medical Journal* **306**: 1115–17.

Hanley I, Cleary E, Oates A and Walker M (1981) In touch with reality. *Social Work Today* **12**(42): 8–10.

Higgs P, MacDonald L and Ward M (1992) Responses to the institution among elderly patients in hospital long-stay care. *Society of Scientific Medicine* **35**(3): 287–93.

Hilgard E, Atkinson R and Atkinson R (1979) *Introduction to Psychology*, 7th edn. New York: Harcourt Brace Jovanovich.

Holden V and Woods R (1982) *Reality Orientation, Psychological Approaches to the Confused Elderly*. London: Churchill Livingstone.

Kelly M (1992) Designing for people with dementia: a review of the literature. In: Coles R *et al.* (1992) *Signposts not Barriers*. Stirling: University of Stirling Dementia Services Development Centre.

Marston N and Gupta H (1977) Interesting the old. *Community Care*, 16 November, 26–28.

Miller E (1977) The management of dementia: a review of some possibilities. *British Journal of Clinical Psychology* **16**: 77–83.

National Health Service and Community Care Act (1990) London: HMSO.

Norman A (1987) *Severe Dementia: The Provision of Long Stay Care*. London: London Centre for Policy on Ageing.

Norman A (1989) *Mental Illness in Old Age: Meeting the Challenge*. London: Centre for Policy on Ageing.

Oddy R and Lodge L (1993) Special support. *Nursing Times* **89**(3): 44–46.

Phair L (1991) Time to let go. *Nursing Times* **87**(35): 27–29.

Phair L and Good E (1989) People not patients. *Nursing Times* **85**(23): 43–44.

Rai G, Stewart K, Van der Cammen T and Veenendall D (1989) Impairment of smell and taste in normal elderly and in patients with Alzheimer's dementia. *Care of the Elderly* **1**(6): 280–81.

Sommer R and Ross H (1958) Social interaction in a geriatric ward. *International Journal of Social Psychiatry* **4**: 128–33.

Stokes G (1988a) *Wandering*. Bicester: Winslow Press.

Stokes G (1988b) *Screaming and Shouting*. Bicester: Winslow Press.

Tothill C (1992) Diary of a carer. *Nursing Times* **18**(47): 34–36.

Wightman A (1992) Provision of a caring environment for people with dementia. Some design principles – an architect's perspective. In: Coles R *et al.* (1992) *Signposts not Barriers*. Stirling: University of Stirling Dementia Services Development Centre.

Wilson-Barnett J (1976) Patients' emotional reactions to hospitalisation. *Journal of Advanced Nursing* **1**: 351–58.

4 Communication
The skill of effective interaction

Difficulties in communication are commonly associated with dementia and older people. The 'problem' is usually perceived as an inherent part of the illness and little is done to compensate for areas of difficulty or to enhance areas of strength. Equally there are important issues regarding how staff communicate with each other, particularly where they work for different organisations. The language used to describe aspects of behaviour, assessments and care is often particular to an establishment or a service and misunderstandings can easily occur when staff need to exchange information on an interagency basis.

In this chapter we will explore these issues and discuss what skills are needed to enable staff to communicate effectively with older people, their carers and other concerned family members.

POINTS TO PONDER

- How much conversation do staff have in your unit with each older person? Do some people appear to 'hog' conversations and do others seem to be excluded? Is most conversation task orientated?

- Do the staff deal consistently with people who are 'deluded'?

- Would the entire staff group agree about the definition of words used to describe 'problem' behaviour, e.g. 'aggressive'?

- Do all staff find care plans useful? How do you ensure that they are regularly read?

- How creative are the staff about using methods of communication other than the spoken word?

- Do other agencies find the information you provide useful and accurate? Have you ever asked them?

- Do staff feel comfortable talking to distressed relatives, do they have appropriate skills? How do you know?

- What do you call the people who use your service? Patients, residents, users? Why? What effect does it have on the philosophy of care?

TALKING TO PEOPLE WITH DEMENTIA

What are the priorities in the care of older people with dementia? People need to be kept safe, warm, comfortable and well nourished and the environment needs to be kept clean and tidy. In some situations it is clear that these tasks consume all the staff's time and energy, thus denying older people the possibility of having their social, emotional and spiritual needs met. Efforts need to be made to care for the 'whole' person and this means acknowledging that older people with dementia have the same, or greater, range of needs as everyone else.

Human beings are social animals and communication between people is fundamental to our survival and well-being. It is hard to imagine a life that does not involve some form of communication, but we have all had experiences in our everyday lives that have been made more or less satisfactory by the quality of communication: think of the frustration and anxiety that used to be induced by the 'hard to decipher' British Rail announcement, or the hurt felt when someone calls you by the wrong name.

It is generally appreciated that people with dementia often have difficulty understanding the world in which they live and making sense of their environment, yet we often seem to imagine that less communication is needed for people with this illness.

> The ordinary human need for social interactions with staff is increased by the fact that old people in homes often have little physical contact with anyone else and because the quality of their interaction with other residents is patchy. (Stevenson 1989)

Where does this belief come from? Does it relate to a fundamental assumption that people with dementia are 'not the same as us' or does it relate more to the difficulty in achieving successful communication with people with dementia? Or is it a reflection of the low priority given to socio-emotional care and the high priority given to the provision of physical care?

There is an acknowledgement that skills involved in verbal communication are frequently affected by the illness but, all too often, older people with dementia are condemned to a world devoid of much of the richness of normal social contact. Kitwood and Bredin (1991) have described the failure of others to treat an individual with dementia with proper attention and respect as contributing more to the destruction of the person than the illness itself.

There is nothing about the illness *per se* that makes people less sociable or less in need of the ordinary conversation and interaction that helps all of us pass the time and make sense of our environment. All too often the communications between staff and older people with dementia relate primarily to practical matters. The tone and content of the conversation may rarely show respect and highlight people's abilities but instead may show disrespect and highlight shortcomings.

In many units the people who are most able and those who are most 'troublesome' get the most attention, the most staff time and the most opportunities for conversation. The people who cause little bother, who sit passively and those who are deemed the most impaired are often ignored for long periods. Without social contact people become withdrawn; people who are withdrawn are not spoken to and so the downward spiral continues.

The quality and content of the conversation is more important than quantity. The verbal content, the tone and speed of the interaction are all important. These variations will transmit additional information to the listener and are usually called 'paralanguage' (Hargie, Saunders and Dickson 1981). The following comment could be said by staff in a kindly way and meant to tease, but could be heard by an older person as pejorative and threatening:

'Fred, what's wrong? You haven't lost your glasses again. You're hopeless, what will we do with you?'

or this, said to encourage action and prevent a wife's distress:

'If you don't put on clean clothes your wife will be ashamed to be seen out with you.'

The style of communication that people use is a reflection of the relationship they have and the esteem, or lack of esteem, that they have for each other. People talk differently to their boss and to the person they employ to fix the plumbing. Staff in the caring professions talk differently to cognitively intact older people and to intellectually impaired older people, in spite of the fact that the intact older person may have been a plumber and the person with dementia may have been a managing director.

The difficulties that people have in talking to people with dementia seem to fall into two broad categories: first there is the person who wants to feel comfortable talking to the older person but does not know 'what to talk about'. This difficulty is usually caused by a lack of sufficient knowledge of the older person and their life. It is much easier to talk to people if we have some idea about their past, their family situation and their interests. This difficulty can be overcome by ensuring that staff are encouraged to 'get to know the person'. Family photographs and scrapbooks can both play an important part as visual clues to the person's past.

The second difficulty that some people may have is more difficult to resolve. They may believe that communicating with people with dementia is a proper use of time when it relates to the giving of instruction or the collection of information but believe that 'conversation' is an inappropriate use of a professional's time. This may be a reflection of negative and ageist attitudes or of a tendency to undervalue older people with dementia. People with this difficulty will rarely admit the problem but will avoid opportunities for conversation. The difficulty will be further manifested by communications often appearing awkward, banal or patronising. The solution lies in the devising of procedures that constantly remind staff that the older people in their care have had full, active and interesting lives. They may need to be reminded that anyone can become demented and that people with dementia should be treated as we ourselves would wish to be treated. They may think that because someone has a memory problem that 'It's not worth talking to them, they won't remember'. If this is the case then they need reminding that most people do things for momentary pleasure, not for the possible pleasant memory.

Some staff may think that managers finding staff talking to older people indicates that they are not 'pulling their weight' and that talking to people can only be done when all the routine tasks have been completed. The managers must ensure that they give clear messages, continually reinforced, that time spent talking to older people is valued. The routine of units should enhance the potential for good care and not over-prioritise domestic tasks at the expense of opportunities for conversation.

Two important features are found in all successful communication. First, it must be timely and secondly, it must be relevant. Effective communication must take place at the right time, be of the right length and be appropriate to the situation. These features apply to communication with older people with dementia and when added to the belief that older people with dementia are of equal value to any other member of society can lead us to establish the following 'rules'.

- Always assume that a person with dementia can understand. Never say anything within the hearing of the person if you do not want them to hear it.

- Use short sentences. This is not to advocate that people are spoken to in 'telegraph English' but rather that sentences should not be so long that the beginning of the sentence is forgotten before the end of the sentence is reached.

- Avoid the use of modern jargon (the hi-fi, 'going to the loo'). Also avoid the use of expressions that should not be taken literally. An example of this would be: 'Come on, jump to it' or 'I'll be just a minute'.

- If you are not understood, be prepared to repeat the question in a different way. Try not to introduce too many new words.

  'Are you hungry, Mrs Smith?'

  'Mrs Smith, would you like something to eat?'

  Or:

  'John, it's Wednesday today, do you want me to get you some shopping?'

  'I'm going to the shops, John, do you want anything?'

  You will notice that in both of these instances the speaker has included the person's name. This simple mechanism is often sufficient to ensure that you capture someone's attention.

- Where you are giving instructions, break down the actions into simple steps. Rather than: 'Mr Anderson, it's time to get dressed', try laying out the clothes in sequence, handing them to Mr Anderson one by one with an appropriate instruction:

  'Here is your vest'

  'Put it on over your head'

- Ensure that you maximise conditions that may improve communication and minimise any distractions. Ensure that the person is comfortable (warm enough; not having an urgent need to go to the toilet) and is wearing their dentures and glasses. Switch off the television or radio. Try to maintain eye contact throughout the conversation. Holding someone's hand while talking to them can be reassuring and help to maintain concentration, but may not always be appropriate.

- Be aware that different people will have different degrees of success in communicating with people. Sometimes this will relate to their appearance; if someone resembles your best friend from your schooldays you will listen to them differently than if they look like a detested head-teacher. Similarly, an older person may find it difficult to take advice from a member of staff who looks younger than their grandchildren.

- Watch for signs of restlessness and withdrawal. Where necessary, tell the person that you understand that it is not a good time to talk and that you will come back later. Make sure that you do return; do not assume that the person will have forgotten.

- Immediate reassurance or reward is important. Reality for some people with dementia is often only in the immediate here and now.

- Try to state things in a positive rather than negative way. Consider the sentence: 'Don't get into the bath with your clothes on'. You only have to miss one word, 'don't', to completely and diametrically alter the meaning of the sentence.

- Try to be relaxed while talking; unnecessary fidgeting or a strident tone can distract from the message.

Television, radio and music must be played at an appropriate volume and it may confuse people if they are used as a continual background noise. Sounds that are half heard are both misleading and frustrating. Similarly, the noise of vacuum cleaners, washing machines and traffic noise may make communication less easy and background noise and echoes can be mis-identified and lead to increased confusion.

Appreciate the importance of both the tone and the volume of your voice. Many older people suffer from some degree of hearing loss; this can be an additional problem for those who have dementia but some basic information about hearing loss will help staff to compensate for this.

Some older people with dementia will have become deaf prior to the onset of the dementia and may be accustomed to wearing a hearing aid. For these people it is important that staff know who wears hearing aids and in which ear they should be fitted. For someone who is confused and forgetful staff will probably have to switch the aid on and off, adjust the volume and identify when a new battery is needed. For those who become deaf after they show signs of dementia it may not be appropriate to consider trying to accustom them to using a hearing aid. They may not tolerate the processes involved in being fitted for a hearing aid and they may not be prepared to keep this 'foreign object' in their ear. New hearing aid users have to learn how to concentrate on key sounds and filter out unwanted or distracting background noise; people with dementia may not be able to do this and may find the sudden magnification of sound distressing.

Staff also need to be aware that for most people with hearing loss particular tones of voice are most easily heard. It may well be that some staff have more success in communicating than others and that this relates to the pitch of their voice. A low tone of voice is often easier to hear. Staff need to appreciate that shouting to someone who is deaf is not helpful and if that person is dementing the shouting may often be mis-interpreted. Older people who are deaf rarely have the same amount of hearing loss in both ears and it is helpful to experiment on which ear is less damaged. There is often merit in ensuring that they do not have excess wax in their ears if they do; a visit to the doctor for 'syringing' may have real benefits.

For some older people with dementia who are substantially confused, the tone of voice may be all that they can focus on. Careful thought needs to be given to how stress, agitation and aggression may be exacerbated by someone's misunderstanding of the tone of voice in which they are addressed. When listening to a conversation in a foreign language and without any knowledge of the language, it is usually possible to ascertain the emotional content of the discussion or at least to distinguish between anger and fright, anxiety and sympathy and caring and control.

UNDERSTANDING AND USING BODY LANGUAGE

We all have a sense of our own private space. Hall (1966) studied man's spatial needs and his work indicates that the extent of personal space with which we each feel comfortable is culturally determined but affected by our social status. In considering the impact of personal space on the provision of care and effective communication, two zones described by Pease (1984) are particularly relevant. He describes an 'intimate zone', the space that is usually only entered by people we are emotionally close to. This zone surrounds us to a depth of 6–18 inches. The 'personal zone' of between 18 and 48 inches describes the distance we stand from each other in most social situations.

The importance of everyone's intimate space needs to be acknowl-edged and staff needing to enter the intimate zone of someone they are caring for need to be aware that it will often be interpreted as either a sexual advance or a hostile action. The 'invasion' should always be accom-panied by an invitation ('nurse, come and help me with my buttons') or by explanation ('I'm just going to brush your hair, Mrs Jones'), other-wise staff run the risk of being repelled either by word, look or action. If any members of a staff group are not convinced about the sense of intrusion that can be felt when someone gets 'too close', we recommend that they experiment for themselves. A comfortable personal space for most people has a radius of at least 24 inches.

The spatial relationship is important. It is no accident that naughty schoolchildren are kept standing by the headmaster's desk, or that friends confiding secrets sit side by side. Many older people receiving care will spend long periods of time in bed or in a chair. Staff should ensure that they do not tower over people. Being on the same level as others can be achieved by sitting on the bed, kneeling alongside their chair or by the managers of the unit investing in settees.

Copstead (1980) was one of the first workers to look at the effects of touch on older people. She hypothesised that an appropriate touch can be an effective manifestation of positive regard. More recently Murphy (1986) has said,

> Communicating by touch is something that we take for granted within our own families and something that elderly people often miss when they have been widowed or ill for a long time or have lived alone without much personal contact.

Skilful use of touch can increase attention and maximise the person's ability to relate and respond to their carer. It can bring comfort and reassurance and a sense of well-being. An older person's feeling of lack of self-worth can be accentuated if the people who care for them seem unwilling to touch them except to carry out physical care tasks. An inappropriate touch may be seen as an invasion and precipitate an aggressive outburst.

NONVERBAL COMMUNICATION

Nonverbal communication includes posture, expression, touch, tone and the spatial relationship of speaker to listener. Some element of nonverbal communication accompanies all verbal communication and can be just as easily misunderstood as words. Think about the movement involved in patting someone's hand reassuringly. The only difference between this and the movement involved in a slap is the force and speed of the action. The importance of nonverbal communication can not be overemphasised. Birtwhistell (1970) claims that the average adult only speaks for 10–11 minutes daily; in the average encounter the verbal element only conveys one-third of the social meaning and nonverbal communication conveys the remaining two-thirds.

Nonverbal communication provides essential feedback to both parties. Not only may an older person with dementia get some sense of meaning from the way the message is given but a carer may find that they can assess how the person they are caring for is feeling and how they are perceiving and understanding the message by looking at their posture or by feeling tension while holding their hand.

Argyle (1967) hypothesised that the sender is often unaware of their nonverbal communication but that it will be plain to the receiver. Argyle also produced a simple but useful diagram:

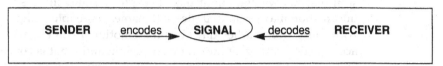

People can learn to be more aware of nonverbal communication and can learn to 'decode' signals from others. Many signals are familiar to us; if we watched people waiting to be interviewed for a job, we could spot the restless fidgeter and the relaxed confident applicant. Books such as that written by Pease (1984) will help staff become more adept at communicating in all kinds of social settings. It is important not to assume that these skills are only useful when communicating with colleagues and the use of nonverbal communication by people with dementia must not be underestimated.

Most of the time nonverbal communication is used to reinforce the spoken message but it can be used to contradict the spoken word. From time to time, we will probably all have said 'Oh, I'm fine' or 'No, I'm not worried', when our facial expression and posture indicate exactly the opposite.

People with dementia may not always be able to identify 'mismatches' in verbal and nonverbal communication. It is thought that in these situations the message behind the nonverbal signals takes precedence (Shapiro 1968; Gravell 1988).

Nonverbal communication is one of the major ways in which feedback on the success of any intervention is given. As people listen to each other, a nod or shake of the head indicates agreement or disagreement while a lack of interest is indicated to the speaker by the breaking off of eye to eye contact, yawning or fidgeting. One of the major difficulties in talking to people with dementia may be the lack of appropriate nonverbal cues that confirm to the speaker that the message has been 'received and understood'. In these situations it is necessary to build into the verbal element of the communication ways of checking how the listener has understood the message.

LISTENING TO OLDER PEOPLE

The conversation of some older people with dementia is often dismissed as 'rubbish' and little effort is made to understand the content of their conversation. Much can be understood, to varying degrees, if one has sufficient knowledge about their background and life history. Often the information may be 'inaccurate' with names of people and places confused with those from earlier days but the emotional content will often be an accurate description of how they are feeling and what is concerning them. Staff need to take time, to listen actively, to pay attention to the language being used and to 'translate' the content into the current contextual framework. The skills required are not that dissimilar to those skills of 'active listening' used in counselling.

> The good listener is an active listener, one truly engaged in the communication process, one who goes out of himself in search of significant cues emitted by others. (Egan 1977)

Effective listening involves having both the time and the inclination. It requires the member of staff to have taken the trouble to find out about the older person and to have the skill to 'decode' information. The effective listener will make an effort to show that they value the person with dementia and that they will treat any information they are given with respect. This can mean making a decision to believe what people with dementia say unless it can be proved to be untrue; in practice, this may mean not assuming that every statement of 'I've been robbed' is an attempt to cover up for a mislaid item, or that a claim of important connections to the aristocracy is fallacious.

WRITTEN COMMUNICATION

Care plans and reports are only effective if they are useable, understood by all staff and accurately reflect situations, problems and behaviours. This requires them to be updated as often as necessary to ensure that they are current and to be written in language that is both readily understood and conveys the appropriate meaning. This is most likely to happen when unspecific, 'shorthand' words such as 'difficult', 'hostile', 'aggressive' are avoided and more specific descriptions used. An example would be to substitute 'may lash out if approached from behind' for 'aggressive'.

It is tempting to use these easy, shorthand terms, but if you do you must take the time to check that all staff understand these words in the same way as you and you must induct new members of staff in their use. Care plans must not be exclusive; they should be available to all members of staff who are likely to come into contact with the person they relate to; the domestic staff, gardener and volunteers may all need to know how to handle situations and may all have different, helpful insights into the person and their behaviour. Care plans should include both short-term and long-term goals and agreed strategies for coping with a variety of possible situations.

Staff and carers frequently ask for reassurance that they are treating appropriately people who appear deluded. They want to know whether it is better to agree, tell the truth or distract them. There is no simple answer but the following scenario may help to clarify the issue.

You are an elderly lady spending 2 weeks in a respite care unit. You normally live at home with your husband. You have dementia. In the unit you are often restless, spending many hours walking the corridors of the unit looking for your mother. The fact that you never find her causes you distress. As you walk around you meet one of the domestic staff. She asks you where you are going and when you explain she laughs and says:

'Good grief, your mum must be 120 by now.'

Around the next corner you meet a student on placement in the unit. You ask him if he has seen your mother. He tells you:

'She is dead, she died in 1956, you ought to go back to the lounge as it's nearly coffee time.'

He points you in the right direction. On your way back to the lounge you meet a volunteer who, seeing that you are distressed, asks you if she can help. You tell her of your difficulty and she tells you that she expects your mother has just popped out for some shopping and will be back later.

The cumulative effect of these interventions will have been to confuse. They may also have destroyed trust and created distress. No one person meant harm but the lack of an appropriate strategy led staff not to act in a therapeutic manner.

Imagine instead that the dialogue with the first member of staff had been:

'Hello how are you?'

'I'm looking for mother, have you seen her?'

'No, but I can see that you are anxious, would you like to stay with me and help me finish this dusting?'

If this first intervention had not worked it would have been important for each subsequent intervention to be conducted along similar lines. The facts are neither denied nor confirmed but the underlying feelings are acknowledged.

Take the case of an elderly man who has come into residential care following the death of this wife. He often forgets why he has to stay. Every time the situation is explained to him it is as if he has heard the news of her death for the first time. Is it appropriate to keep on reminding him or should the staff find some other reason to explain his presence there? There is no single answer that can be prescribed. Instead, the staff group should look at creative solutions and strategies and all agree to implement them. Ideas that may be helpful include the compiling of a scrapbook about his wife, or staff assisting him to write a diary of recent events that can be kept and read frequently.

The value of written material should not be underestimated. The ability to write and to understand the written word appears not to be totally dependent on the ability to speak and understand the spoken word. Where there are difficulties in communicating by speech it is always worth writing the message down, making sure that your handwriting is both legible and large enough. The length of the person's concentration span may be short but notes and simple instructions may have their uses. There are occasions when written material is particularly important. Someone receiving respite care may be worried and constantly searching for their carer. A letter or postcard in their pocket or handbag may assist in their understanding of the situation. Staff may need to prompt people to look for the message and read it but there will often be more comfort in recognised handwriting than in any amount of reassurance from a stranger. In some situations a diary can help someone to keep track of the days and it is a socially acceptable way of keeping useful information to hand.

For people being cared for at home labels on doors and cupboards may help to preserve orientation. A list of commonly needed telephone numbers can be posted by the telephone, a note can be stuck to the freezer plug saying 'Do not unplug'. Similarly, people may find it reassuring to have a written programme of weekly activities and anticipated visitors, as shown in the example below.

Monday	5 May	9 a.m.	Bus collects for the day centre – take £1.00 for lunch.
Tuesday	6 May	9 a.m.	Home help – Mary.
Wednesday	7 May	9 a.m.	Day centre, bus comes at 9. £1.00 for lunch. Bath day.
Thursday	8 May	11 a.m.	Home help – will collect pension and do shopping.
Friday	9 May	3 p.m.	Appointment at GPs. Sally to take you.

Saturday 10 May 12.30 p.m. Mrs Jones bringing lunch in for you.

Sunday 11 May 11.30 a.m. Son coming to take you to lunch.

COMMUNICATING WITH RELATIVES

Staff often need to talk to relatives and carers to ascertain information, elicit views and to make assessments about a person's ability to offer appropriate care. The subject matter involved in these discussions is sensitive and the context of the discussions is often one of fraught and emotional circumstances. Staff need to be aware of the potential range of feelings of the relatives and carers and the mixed emotions often involved in caring. Where discussions relate to the future care of the person with dementia staff should be aware that family members may be grateful for some offer of help but concerned about the impact of losing control and being dependent on a statutory agency. They may be pleased to be supported in the caring role but angry and guilty at having to acknowledge that their care is no longer sufficient.

Staff need to be aware of the family dynamics and the history of the caring relationship. Members of staff must take care not to overlay the situation with their assumptions of how the family behaved and what family members will prefer and desire.

Careful thought should be given about the information collected when someone is admitted to a unit, or care at home is being negotiated. Families are obvious and useful sources of information about daily routines. Carers should be encouraged to write down this information and include their relative's preferences. This can then form the core of a care plan. Families may need assistance in order to understand the kind of information you would find useful. This information is best organised and exchanged well before admission or the commencement of a service, both these being stressful events. Staff should also ensure that family members have written information about how to contact the unit or community staff's office and the best time to telephone.

In units offering day care thought should be given to how messages and information are relayed between staff and carer. These could range from a message from the unit about an outing to a request for information about a sudden change in mobility. In most cases a written message is required; in some establishments a staff member accompanies the day centre's users home on the centre's minibus and can take this opportunity to collect and deliver information. Many carers comment on their curiosity about how the person they care for acts in the centre, what they eat, what they talk about and how they spend their day. They would value the opportunity to ask and see what happens. For many of them the only chance they have to talk to staff is during assessment or pending discharge or at a review and they may feel that any of these are too important a meeting to 'waste time' asking questions that may appear trivial. Thought should be given to ways of enabling key workers to have contact with carers to allow informal feedback. Other, more creative, options are available to staff; in one day centre a video was made of a woman who had dementia enjoying a swimming session. She had been a keen and able swimmer and the short video, although showing her needing a great deal of assistance, was highly valued by her family. The woman rarely spoke or showed pleasure but while swimming was both relaxed and smiling.

Where there is a large and extended family it may be helpful for the family to nominate one person to be the main channel for communication. This can both cut down on the number of calls to a unit to check that someone is all right and can ensure that all family members receive the same information. If this is arranged it is vital that staff know to contact the named person and that the named person always lets the unit know when they are unavailable and nominates a substitute.

Many friends, families and carers find visiting someone with dementia difficult and stressful. The situation can be eased if staff have ensured that visitors feel able to assist in the care or if there are activities to hand that they can join in with the person they are visiting. Staff can also assist by ensuring that different people's visitors are introduced to each other. In some units this will lead to people taking an interest in someone else's relative while the visitors are on holiday, or may encourage them to visit more frequently because of the companionship they find. Relatives can often find comfort in shared experiences and solutions for each other's difficulties.

Family Language

In every family there are real or invented words that have special meanings and in addition there are differences between geographical regions and between social classes. Staff need to clarify the use of such coded language, particularly where it relates to the provision of care or the expression of feelings and emotions. Examples of these codes could be words like 'cack' meaning 'left' to some people and 'excrement' to others; 'mithered' meaning confused and worried or cold, depending on where you were brought up. People who do not have English as their first language may revert during the course of the illness to their mother tongue.

There will be occasions where translation skills are required. Perhaps the relatives could teach the staff a few words of the language, the most essential being, 'please speak English, I do not understand French/Greek/Urdu, etc.'

In residential units visitors will often be dependent on staff to find out what has happened since their last visit and will usually rely on staff to provide information about the person's health. It may be that the person has dramatically improved since admission and staff need to understand the effect that this news may have on someone who may have spent years looking after the person, perhaps to the detriment of their own health. The person's health or behaviour may have deteriorated since admission; the news of this may unleash hostility and anger or relief that 'no one can care as they do'.

Wherever professional staff are involved in the care of older people with dementia they will be perceived as experts by friends and family members, many of whom will be hungry for information about the illness. Careful consideration needs to be given to how news is told, how much information is given at any one time and the language used. The goal is to share an understanding of the illness honestly and gradually, with the family setting the pace. On occasions the family will include children or teenagers. Special care must be taken to give them appropriate information. An increasing number of people, these days, have some idea about the nature of the illness, many will have particular concerns about how the disease will affect them and need to explore with you issues relating to theories about the role of genetics in the illness and the expectations that staff will have about families' willingness and ability to provide care. These are areas of concern for most families and carers; some carers will find it difficult to admit that they want to be relieved of the burden of care, some will want to discuss issues surrounding the prolonging of life, for instance by the use of antibiotics in infections. Others may want to disclose real or potential abuse. Each member of staff should be equipped with appropriate skills to enable relatives to talk openly about these difficult issues. Staff members will need to be non-judgemental and gently encouraging.

COMMUNICATING WITH COLLEAGUES AND OTHER AGENCIES

Words can have very different meanings depending on the environment in which you work, your professional training and your own value base. For professionals to work well together they need to be clear about each other's use of language. All too often people are embarrassed or think that colleagues are too busy to ask for clarification and discrepancies only become apparent when there are problems. Words come to mean different things to different people. A prime example of this can be demonstrated by looking closer at the use of the words 'incontinent' and 'wandersome'.

Imagine Mrs Wright, an 80-year-old woman describing a problem faced by her while caring for her demented husband. She tells the district nurse that he is wandersome and has started being incontinent. The same gentleman begins attending a day centre and staff report that he 'escaped' twice during the first day but was not incontinent. He is admitted to a general ward of a hospital for treatment of a chest infection and the ward sister tells Mrs Wright that her husband was incontinent and only just mobile. The differences in how he appears in different settings could be explained by fluctuations in the illness or could be explained by having the following information.

Mr Wright lives in a small terraced house, cluttered with furniture and four cats. He used to be a man who rarely took exercise and relied on his wife to 'fetch and carry' for him. He now follows her wherever she goes, although he only walks a few yards at a time; this change in behaviour causes her great distress. His incontinence is caused by her changing the colour of the paintwork on the toilet door. He used to know that the blue door led to the toilet. In the day centre he can identify the toilet by its clearly marked sign. He leaves in an effort to find his wife.

In the general hospital, Mr Wright is incontinent because the toilets are out of sight and no one has reminded him recently of their whereabouts. He walks just as far as he did at home but in a ward 30 yards long it causes difficulty.

This is a relatively simple example; consider the range of possible interpretations in the following: aggressive, disinhibited, antisocial, dirty . . . to make sense of each we need to know a great deal more about the circumstances, values, experience and attitudes of the person using the word.

The medical and nursing professions, perhaps more than social services, have a plethora of technical terms. Most have an exact definition and are used to describe symptoms, illnesses and treatments. Staff from other professional groups must not be afraid to ask for clarification and explanation. Nursing and medical staff should make it easy for others to ask and not try to mystify their profession. In any team each member should respect and understand how their colleagues use language.

Between teams of people who regularly work together or 'share' clients (district nurses/home helps) or refer people to each other's service (ward sister/day centre manager) there needs to be a clear understanding of the trigger words each may use. What does 'urgent', 'particularly vulnerable' and 'high priority' mean for each agency? Staff also need to be aware of the code words used to describe certain difficult aspects of situations. Each staff group needs to understand how terminal illness may be described in the case notes of someone who is unaware of the diagnosis; or how suspected abuse or the potential for abuse is noted.

Much business today is conducted over the telephone and it is far easier to 'get the wrong end of the stick' over the telephone than in face to face communication. This is usually because we lack visual clues to assist our understanding and are forced to rely on the content and tone of the message, with minimal opportunities for seeking clarification or giving feedback.

For those centres receiving referrals from the public or taking telephone calls from carers, special thought needs to be given to the telephone manner of all the staff. Imagine a carer concerned about their relative, or someone who has finally gathered the courage to ring and ask for help. If either of these people's telephone calls are dealt with carelessly great damage can be done. It could be assumed that the unit is poorly run simply by the way their call is handled. Carers can lose heart and confidence and decide not to ask for advice or help. There needs to be an agreed formula for what is said when the telephone is answered and a policy on how messages are taken. A quality service will also appreciate that a telephone left unanswered for a period of time gives an unfortunate impression. Someone ringing may, in theory, understand that the telephone is not being answered because staff are attending to the urgent needs of people resident in the unit, but in reality are still likely to conjure up an image of staff sitting around drinking coffee.

The image and credibility of many services relies to a large extent on word of mouth. Major catering chains work on the assumption that consumers tell three people about a good experience but 10 people about a bad experience. Given that older people increasingly may have a choice of service, particularly in residential care settings, it is vital for the continuing success of any unit that it is 'marketable'. Where market forces or statutory fee rates have ensured that most units charge similar fees the value of the unit's image can not be overemphasised. The telephone manner of the staff, the impression given by brochures and the 'word of mouth' factor become keys to continued success.

GIVING FEEDBACK

Communication skills become of prime importance when we consider the need to be able to either praise or correct the way care is being delivered, whether by staff member or family carer. In many settings there is little encouragement to comment positively on care, attitudes or endeavours. The emphasis is often on criticising 'bad' care practices and more time and effort is allocated to reprimand rather than commend. The morale of a staff team or of a carer can be visibly improved by managers and professionals taking time to ensure that they communicate their approval effectively. In a unit it is immensely helpful if an atmosphere can be created where each member of staff finds the time and the words to commend good practice.

ACTION FOR CHANGE

1. Consider the benefits of auditing the communication systems in your establishment as it affects older people. A good starting point may be to analyse the patterns of conversation in the lounge. Spend an hour or two observing who says what to whom and why. Are there areas where practice could be improved?

2. To improve written communication introduce a system of fines; first compile, with your colleagues, a list of words that you find unhelpful: 10p is put into a charity box every time someone uses one.

3. Set standards for the way the telephone will be answered. An example may be: within six rings, with the staff member saying, 'Good morning/afternoon/evening, Parkview Home, can I help you?' Monitor the standards by getting someone to ring in regularly and report on the experience.

4. Devise a simple way of asking colleagues if the written information you give them is acceptable. If you frequently compile 'continuation of care' forms for community based staff, consider asking them to return one form a week with comments about its usefulness.

5. Look at the written material your unit uses. Is it current and attractive? Ask carers for their views. If they report that it could be improved do something about it. If you have a relatives' support group attached to your unit why not ask them to write it?

6. Where possible provide opportunities for the whole staff team together to examine issues relating to communication. Work out some simple exercises that will highlight areas of strength and weakness (Evans and Hind 1987).

REFERENCES

Argyle M (1967) *The Psychology of Interpersonal Behaviour.* Harmondsworth: Penguin.

Birtwhistell R L (1970) *Kinesics and Context.* Philadelphia: University of Pennslyvania Press.

Copstead L (1980) Effects of touch on self appraisal and interaction appraisal for permanently institutionalised older adults. *Journal of Gerontological Nursing* 6(12): 747.

Egan G (1977) In: Stewart J (ed.) *Listening as Empathic Support. Bridges not Walls.* Reading, Massachusetts: Addison–Wesley.

Evans K and Hind T (1987) Getting the message across. *Nursing Times* 83(18): 40–42.

Gravell R (1988) *Communication Problems in Elderly People. Practical Approaches to Management.* London: Croom Helm.

Hall E T (1966) *The Hidden Dimension.* New York: Doubleday & Co.

Hargie O, Saunders C and Dickson D (1981) *Social Skills in Interpersonal Communication.* London: Croom Helm.

Kitwood T and Bredin K (1991) *Person to Person. A Guide to the Care of Those With Failing Mental Powers.* Bradford: Gale Centre Publications.

Murphy E (1986) *Dementia and Mental Illness in the Old.* London: Papermac.

Pease A (1984) *Body Language. How to Read Others' Thoughts by their Gestures.* London: Sheldon Press.

Shapiro J G (1968) Responsivity to facial and linguistic cues. *Journal of Communication.* **18**: 11–17.

Stevenson O (1989) *Age and vulnerability: A guide to better care. Age Concern Handbook.* London: Edward Arnold.

5 The Day around the Person

How routines make or break positive approaches to care

People in institutions live in groups that are not of their choosing and as a consequence of their admission will have suffered separation from their family and familiar surroundings. How people experience life within an institution can dramatically affect their mental health and level of functioning. Most institutions have daily and weekly routines bedded in their history and the notion of institutionalisation is based on the proposition that damage is done to people by overriding their personal wishes by enforced routines. Are routines always damaging and are they inevitable? When does a routine become a ritual? Is it possible to let people with dementia live their lives exactly as they wish?

People with dementia living at home may be subjected to other people's routines. The advent of the Community Care Act will mean that more people are supported at home and there is a danger that the visits of numerous 'visitors' offering a service may impose their own routines and destroy the person's remaining individualised life style.

The organisation of the day, both within an institution and the community, can be the vital component in creating a positive environment or a disempowering prison.

POINTS TO PONDER

- What time of the day do you get up? Do you get up at the same time on your day off?

- Does your unit operate an 'off-duty system' or a 'duty rota'? What difference could this make to the staff's attitudes to work?

- Does your unit have a locked front door? When did you last review the necessity for this?

- How does sleeping in a strange room affect the quality of your rest?

- When do you normally bathe or shower? Could you maintain this pattern if you were a resident in your unit?

- Think about the crockery used in your unit. Do the staff use different crockery to the residents? If so why?

- How do you feel when you have to wait in all day for the gas man to call?

- How often do you enjoy eating your meal in front of the television. How often are people in your unit allowed to do this?

THE BODY'S NATURAL ROUTINE

Contemporary opinion of residential care often ridicules any routines or rituals within the staff daily practice. It is frowned on to 'allow' residents to sit in the same chair every day or for them to claim areas or pieces of furniture as their own. Any ensuing squabbles may be sorted out by the staff taking the parent role and reinforcing the notion that no one has the right to claim the same personal space each day. Routines are natural; all of us are institutionalised within our own life experience and some elements of each person's routine will be outside their control. Most people undertake the same tasks each morning as they prepare for the day ahead: we dress, wash and eat in an order and style determined by personal preference, but the time we spend on these actions may well be dictated by the time our employer has decided we should start work.

Many physical and natural processes are governed by the body's own clock, known as a circadian rhythm. The natural body routine seems to be longer than the solar day by 1 hour. In experiments where people are isolated from their normal environment and given no clues about the time of day, the body reverts eventually to a 25-hour day with the pattern of sleep and wakefulness seeming to be dictated by the length of daylight (Totterdell, Smith and Folkard 1992). It is thought that circadian rhythm is controlled by the pineal gland in the hypothalamus, which secretes serotonin. The gland can become calcified with age (Lumley, Craven and Aitken 1980) but the consequences of this are not clear. It is speculated that it may affect the body clock and that abnormalities in the release of serotonin may cause a disturbance in the sleep/wake pattern.

In everyday life, humans do not rely exclusively on their body clock to govern their daily routines; apart from clocks telling us the time there are a wide range of social cues giving indications about the time or the day of the week; the sound of birdsong, church bells, heavy traffic on the road outside or a signature tune on the radio will be familiar cues for many people. A change to the routine, such as the postman calling later than normal, can cause momentary confusion in the most mentally alert.

Another biological phenomenon which is thought to affect everyone is biorhythm. Some people believe that human temperament and behaviour follow predictable persistent patterns which recur over a number of days. As each biorhythm travels through its positive and negative phases it affects how someone copes with life emotionally, physically and intellectually.

Routines would appear to be an integral part of human behaviour and to have routines within an institution or community service is inevitable if chaos is to be avoided. The challenge is how to develop routines that are flexible enough to accommodate each individual's personal systems and to ensure that the routines exist to serve the best interests of the residents rather than the sole interests of the staff group.

Carers at home often report that having a routine assists the person with dementia to make sense of their day and community staff visiting to offer help and support should try, wherever possible, to fit in with this routine. It will be appreciated that when someone with dementia is offered residential respite or day care it makes sense to try to mimic the routines they were familiar with at home. There is an inevitable conflict when several people with dementia are being cared for in a group but it is possible, with thoughtfulness and careful planning, to ensure that each person's routine is changed as little as possible.

THE ROUTINE OF THE NIGHT

The night is often considered to be the quiet time of the day, when least happens. Everyone has a routine for the night time. The phrases 'being an early bird' or 'a night owl' are based on the fact that people are aware that they perform better at some times of day and adjust their lifestyle accordingly. Yet there is a common assumption, on which much institutional routine is based, that all older people like to go to bed early and wake early and that having 'breakfast in bed' is a treat.

Many people have routines and rituals that help them unwind before retiring to bed; they are very individual and may be practised for many years, becoming entrenched into their lifestyle. When a person dements it is recognised that long-term memory and overlearned behaviour remain intact the longest and it is important to consider how care can best be provided in such a way as to recognise, accept and maintain these habits.

The night shift in most institutions is often regarded as the shift people choose to work if they have family commitments or want to maximise their earnings. Many homes have long lists of domestic chores for night staff to undertake and in some units staff have 'permission' to sleep if it is not busy. Notoriously night staff are offered, and take up, fewer training opportunities than day staff and they are infrequently involved in decision making arenas. They are often not offered supervision and remain isolated from the day staff. There are coherent arguments made, particularly by managers, that all staff should rotate through both day and night shifts (Walsh and Ford 1989). While this would improve the integration of night and day staff it might prove unpopular with staff and severely disadvantage working women with children.

Regardless of how night staff are organised there is much a unit can do to ensure that its routines are helpful for the majority of residents. As a starting point it is worth considering what time people are 'put to bed'. Is it a reflection of their preferences and needs or related more to the time the night shift comes on duty?

People are given milky drinks at 7.30 p.m. to help them sleep more easily. If people are encouraged to settle down for the night at 7.30 p.m. by giving them external clues that it is bed time, by getting them undressed ready for bed and giving them a night-time drink it is hardly surprising that some people then are wide awake at 6.00 a.m. or earlier. Older people need less sleep than younger people. It would seem more appropriate to encourage older people to stay up until later in the evening and offer the drink and assistance with undressing at a bed-time hour that fits in with their premorbid behaviour.

Many care professionals still take out people's dentures at night and soak them in a denture solution; yet not all older people take their teeth out, some may only remove the upper or the lower set and if this personal routine is disturbed they may become agitated or show 'searching' behaviour. People will also have different routines relating to when and how they wash, yet most establishments have a set routine to which everyone is expected to conform.

Even when people are able to go to bed at their own chosen time a wide range of things may disturb them. The furniture may cast unusual shadows, causing illusions, noises may be unfamiliar, the heating in the bedrooms may be different to what people are used to at home and the bed may be substantially harder or feel different because it has waterproof covers. The sleep pattern of people usually becomes more disturbed as they get older; they may wake naturally because of the need to micturate, because of cramps, dyspnoea or pain (Irwin 1992). If night staff are constantly touring the unit, opening and closing doors and making unnecessary noise they can make someone's sleep pattern even more disturbed. The need to ensure that people are safe must be balanced against the need to try to provide the optimum conditions for a good night's sleep.

Until recently the vast majority of accommodation for people with dementia was in traditional Nightingale wards or multibedded rooms. There was a belief that people with dementia would sleep more soundly with 'company', that if they woke in the night and saw someone else asleep in the room they would be disinclined to wander. This hypothesis takes no account of the fact that some older people may be so alarmed to wake and find a stranger in their bedroom that they would become distressed. An increasing number of units are now offering single rooms and find that many people with dementia value the privacy and quiet.

The night-time toileting routine will also affect how much people are disturbed. Incontinence aids and absorbent sheeting can reduce the amount of direct handling a person will need. The continence assessment process should have taken account of a whole 24-hour period and should provide information to allow for enuresis to be dealt with appropriately throughout the night.

POSITIVE NIGHT CARE IN THE RESIDENTIAL SETTING

Caring at night for people with dementia is often fraught with difficulties. Some organisation and structure is needed to give stability to those people who have enough awareness to distinguish the time of day. What can be done to offer a more positive experience at night?

The shift change should be at a time most appropriate for the people resident in the unit; often the arrival of night staff will be a reminder to some people that it is bedtime. The bed-time drinks should be available just before people retire to bed, rather than be the last task automatically undertaken by the day shift.

At the point of admission a full history should be taken that includes the night-time sleep pattern and the preferred evening routine. If the staff group can replicate this as closely as possible it will increase the chance of a good night's sleep. The preferred times for going to bed and rising should be clearly recorded in the care plan and each person should have an accurate assessment of the enuresis, of any pain and their anxiety and confusion. This should be undertaken by a qualified and experienced care professional.

The fundamental philosophy that will ensure good management at night is that people with dementia should be empowered to find their own balance between activity and wakefulness, rest and sleep, provided this does not pose a health risk either to themselves or others. The care professionals should adapt the needs of the unit around them, ensuring that they do not inflict their own standards on the people in their care (Kelley and Lakin 1988). The same skills and techniques that staff use during the day time are equally useful at night; using diversion to stop ruminations, using slow clear simple instructions and giving people time. Staff should be able to allow people as much expression of choice and control over their nights as over their days. If people choose to sleep in their clothes or not get completely undressed, night staff should always ask themselves, 'Does it really matter?' This question can only be answered by assessing the consequences of the actions on the person, their family and the other residents.

Often the reason for admission of the older person is because the carer can no longer cope with a disturbed sleep pattern. When trying to rectify someone's disturbed sleep pattern it is necessary to take into account physical, environmental and social factors. Where sedatives are being used their efficacy should be monitored by the careful use of a sleep chart.

It has to be appreciated that as dementia progresses there may be changes in the sleep pattern that are difficult or impossible to alter. In a continuing care setting staff must examine their own attitudes and develop a positive philosophy on how this will be handled. Night and day staff must work as a team in order to eliminate any resolvable problems that may be affecting the person's sleep; this will include monitoring the amount of 'cat napping', looking at the amount of mental stimulation and physical exercise and considering if the timing of medication is appropriate. The bed should be comfortable and be positioned in the room to suit each individual, there should be a choice of types of bedding available and a clear-faced, readable clock should be available (Seymour and Bayer 1993). It should be possible for people to bring their own beds into long-term settings even if the mattress needs to be replaced in order to conform to fire regulations. People's sleep may be affected by the proximity of the bed to the toilet, the noises made by other residents and their previous work experiences; a milkman or a shift worker will have a different experience of a normal night's sleep.

Night care in residential settings is no less important than the care given in the day time; the skill, experience and qualifications of the staff should be no less than that of the day staff.

THE NIGHT IN THE COMMUNITY

Where a person with dementia is living at home and is showing disturbed sleep patterns it may be more difficult for the problem to be ameliorated. The 'treatment' will lie in the hands of the carer who should be given all the necessary relevant information about the factors that affect sleep. In many cases the assessment of the problem and advice about management from a community psychiatric nurse will be advantageous and will help to ease tensions. Extended care or night nursing teams are faced with the difficulties of working within limited resources and this can affect the amount of choice an individual can have over the time they go to bed; yet the consequences of putting to bed too early someone who has sleep disturbances must be considered seriously. Schemes such as this must begin to examine ways of being able to operate at times suitable for the client and the carer.

Carers may benefit from night respite. Respite care is traditionally offered in blocks of 1 week or 2 weeks, when the person is taken into a care setting. Innovative schemes are now in operation where a person with a poor sleep pattern can be taken from their home into a care setting only at night time, allowing the carer to have a good night's sleep and the person with dementia to be cared for and assessed by care professionals (Gaze 1990). Night sitting services are also available within the home from some private and voluntary agencies, including St John Ambulance Association, the Red Cross and Crossroads. The funding of these services should be available from Community Care budgets. To be without sleep will cause the carer to feel unable to cope; the effect of a person's sleep pattern on the carer must always be dealt with positively and effectively if the carer is to be able to continue.

THE EARLY MORNING

Many units change shifts from night to day at an early hour. Some night staff, in an attempt to assist their day-time colleagues, will attempt to get people up and dressed before they go off duty. Sometimes they will justify this by saying that 'someone was wet at 6.00 a.m. so it was just as easy to dress them as change the bed linen'.

The potentially heavier workload that faces day staff often means that some things are done by night staff that should be undertaken later in the day. In some establishments night staff are expected not only to get people up and breakfasted before they leave but also dispense the first medicine round of the day, despite the dangers of having medicine being dispensed by tired staff (Walsh and Ford 1989). Limited numbers of drugs should be given before breakfast and these should be only those drugs where the doctor has specifically asked for the drug to be administered at this specific time.

While it is the habit of some units to get everyone up by 7.00 a.m. for breakfast, other units prefer to 'encourage' everyone to have a lie-in and take their breakfast in bed. The enforced lie-in may cause anxiety to those people who were used to getting up early to do their chores or go to work. Although they may not have had to rise early for many years a proportion of older people prefer to continue to get up early. Every person's waking routine should be known to the staff and honoured and supported as far as is possible. Any change or disruption to the routine should be considered and planned and staff should be aware that anxiety levels may increase.

THE HANDOVER

Shift times are often regimented throughout an organisation and are determined by economic factors. Long afternoon overlaps are slowly disappearing and the handover time is becoming more manageable. At the other extreme there are residential settings where staff are expected to transfer information about 24 residents in as little as 15 minutes. The timing of the shifts should reflect the nature of the unit and the length and type of handover should be conducive to the effective and efficient exchange of information. The traditional method of handover involves the senior care professional giving a summary of information to some members, usually the more senior, of the incoming team. The person giving the information may not have been directly involved in any care provision, making the information 'secondhand'. Equally the information may be received by someone who may not be providing care, establishing ideal conditions for poor communication (Walsh and Ford 1989).

There is a trend within health settings towards conducting handovers 'around the bedside', that is, directly between small groups of staff. This means that not all of the patients are discussed with all of the staff and has the advantage of allowing more than one patient to be discussed at a time (Walsh and Ford 1989). This method may not be directly appropriate to settings providing care for people with dementia. In most care situations people with dementia are free to wander and may, during any shift, interact with any member of staff; thus it is imperative that all staff are aware of current treatment, issues and management tactics. A typical scenario in many units will be the 87-year-old person with dementia who constantly seeks her mother. When she asks staff for assistance in this task it is essential that all staff respond consistently. The damaging alternative is that staff responses may vary from the 'don't worry, she'll be here soon' to the 'have you forgotten again, she's dead'.

ALLOCATING THE WORK

Any caring professional working either in an institution or in the community must balance the needs and wishes of individuals with the needs and routines of their organisation, its other customers and their colleagues.

Task Allocation

During the last 15 years there has been intense discussion about the best way of organising work within a care setting. The traditional method of allocating work was undertaken at the beginning of each shift with each care professional being given a job – toiletting, putting away the laundry or making the drinks. This produced a factory-like environment, with the people in the unit becoming items to be processed. In addition this kind of task allocation often took no account of staff members' talents and skills and did not facilitate the learning of new skills. Many care professionals still feel that working through a list of jobs is the most efficient method of getting through the work in spite of the fact that it often provides staff with little job satisfaction. The method is thought to have been popular with the nursing profession because of its similarities with the organisation of the army and was viewed as the best use of human resources. The impact on nursing was to remove the most qualified and experienced nurses away from client contact. Tasks such as bathing and feeding were seen as basic tasks and given to the most junior staff members (Pearson 1988).

The Team Approach

By the 1970s team care had become popular in nursing. This method of staff organisation identified a team of staff led by a qualified practitioner that had a responsibility to plan and deliver care to a specific group of people. It ensured that the older person and their family could build a relationship with staff, there was consistency of approach and the possibility of better supervision of untrained staff (Kron 1976). This approach is commonly found in Social Service establishments and the private and voluntary sectors; it allows staff to develop expertise and focus on individual clients' problems, ensuring a more specialised care strategy for the client. This approach relies on effective team selection, team building and team support and all team members and the team leader must allocate time and effort to looking after the team and dealing promptly with interpersonal issues.

Key Working on a Daily Basis

A popular alternative to task allocation is key working, where each older person is allocated to a member of staff for the duration of a shift. The staff member then has responsibility for this person although the final responsibility for planning care lies with the senior qualified professional. In small establishments this can work well, but is not usually satisfactory in large establishments where the older person may be allocated a different worker each day, denying them the opportunity to build a relationship with their care worker. Where this system is operated great care must be taken that some individuals are not identified as 'problem patients' and always allocated to the newest or most junior member of staff.

Key Working or Primary Care

The language of health and social care professionals varies but the intention and the philosophy behind key working and primary nursing is the same. The difference originated not only from the different titles used in each profession but also as a result of the lack of qualified staff working in social care settings for older people. In nursing a primary nurse must be a qualified first-level nurse, whereas in social care settings the key worker will often have no relevant formal qualification but will be judged competent through experience. Within this system of care the primary nurse or the designated key worker is responsible for the total care of the older person, including assessment and the planning, implementing and evaluation of the care plan. They would also be responsible for negotiating and supporting the family and requesting specialist advice when appropriate. The key worker/primary nurse also carries out direct care and is able to monitor closely the changes in the older person (Wright 1990).

Working alongside them is an associate nurse or care worker who carries out the care designed by the primary nurse in their absence. In health care settings a primary nurse accepts responsibility to facilitate the care of a client and is accountable for their care. The nurse's main function will often be as enabler and negotiator and there is obvious scope to develop both empowering and advocate roles (Black 1992). These are areas that other schemes of delegation can not address. The system has the further advantage of ensuring that new and inexperienced staff work alongside experienced staff and are shown what to do rather than receiving only verbal instruction.

In social care settings the system may be less clear cut given the scarcity of care workers with qualifications. Managers of establishments and organisations may have to devise ways of judging a staff member's competency in order for them to be able to take on the role and responsibilities of a key worker. In many local authority settings there has been a move, over the last 5 years, away from manual grade staff as care assistants to officer grade staff as care officers and the recent national negotiations about the grading of residential staff may clarify the position further.

Some nurses are offended by the linking of the key worker and primary nurse schemes. In their eyes the two roles are not equal and trying to equate them erodes the value of the qualified nurse. The two professional groups need to work ever closer and a recognition of the similarities and differences between the two groups is vital to generate a greater opportunity for constructive collaboration. Staff in social settings have been equally guilty in denying the need for qualified nursing staff in units for people with dementia. Few people today would support the medical model as the best formula for the care of people with dementia; in the appreciation of a more social and homelike way of care some have forgotten the value of the nursing perspective.

THE DUTY ROTA

When staff work should reflect when they are needed in order to offer the optimum care to the older person. This is a noble intention that takes no account of the needs of the worker who may have child care arrangements to make or calligraphy classes to attend on Tuesdays. The duty rota should therefore be a compromise, as unhappy staff and low staff morale will not enhance a positive approach to care delivery. Principles can be adhered to but staff need to be flexible. If the philosophy of primary care or team work is adopted the duty rota must be completed in such a way that every client has one of 'their' workers on duty at all times. Staff need to feel valued and have a flexible duty rota that allows for a personal life.

The rota should be available long enough in advance to ensure that staff can plan their private lives (Walsh and Ford 1989). It must be emphasised that the rota is a duty rota and not an off-duty rota and that the staff have a responsibility to care for the client group and fulfil their obligations to their employer.

Every establishment needs a mechanism to ensure adequate staff cover. In Social Service establishments and the private sector this has often taken the form of agency staffing, which while cost-effective has the disadvantage of providing unfamiliar staff. In hospital settings there has usually been an opportunity to establish a 'bank' of casual staff, each of whom will be familiar with the unit.

Toiletting Routines

Some years ago it was common practice in units caring for people with dementia for all to be toiletted at the same time. In some units this meant queues outside the toilet areas, in others it meant a bathroom with several toilets in it. There was a prevalent belief that people could be 'trained' to empty their bladders at fixed times but the majority of people would be 'padded up' in case of accidents. Good practice now requires that an assessment is made over a 24-hour period that examines a person's normal pattern of voiding. As a result of this assessment an individual care plan should be drawn up and specific aids selected that will assist in the maintenance of continence. Every residential unit and day centre should have access to a range of incontinence aids; a single type of pad will not suit all people. Each staff group should also be aware of the services offered by the local continence adviser and should know how and when to make a referral to this service. It is not acceptable practice to cover all chair seats with incontinence pads 'just in case' and catheterisation should only be considered as a last resort. There is often an assumption that the majority of people in a unit will be incontinent and seating and flooring will be designed with this in mind. The chairs may have waterproof covers, in spite of the fact that no one would have furniture like this in their own home, and the floor covering may be vinyl. A more positive approach would be to assume that with staff assistance most people can be continent and that there is no need for either waterproof chairs or flooring. Obviously, some accidents are inevitable but modern cleaning techniques mean that surfaces are easier to keep clean and odour-free. Surely it is preferable to give older people with dementia the dignity of carpeted floors and comfortable chairs and to face the risk of having occasionally to replace a soiled item.

DRUG ROUNDS

The ritual of the drug round is well developed, particularly in nursing units. The paraphernalia associated with the dispensing of medicines has not changed over the years and in many units all other activity stops while the ritual is in progress. There is status in being permitted to undertake this task and it is rightly seen as a job needing skill and concentration. In other types of units the rules associated with the dispensing of drugs may be less regulated by professional dictate but equally formalised. There are ways of making the routine less intrusive; the medicine should always be taken to the person and not vice versa, trays of medicine should not be carried around public areas and medicine should be stored in small containers that relate to individuals, not as 'stock medication'. Night-time medication can be kept in a locked drawer in each person's bedroom and consideration should be given to the use of monitored dosage systems.

It may be possible for some people to continue to be responsible for their own medication with minimum supervision; for example, they may be able to cope with a single day's drugs. People living in their own home present particular problems and risks: in spite of monitored dosage systems and specially designed pill boxes there may be no alternative but to ensure that a member of the community staff visit every time medicine is required.

BATHING

Helping older people with dementia take a bath is a labour-intensive task. In some units it is necessary to limit the number of baths that any individual has and organise the timing of baths in such a way as to coincide with times when sufficient staff are available: hence the weekly bath, taken in the late morning or early afternoon and the bath book to ensure that everyone gets their turn. Bathing should be not only a necessary routine but a pleasurable time. In order to achieve this it is worth considering the various aspects of washing and bathing that are matters for personal preference. Some people in their 70s and 80s have only ever been used to a weekly bath, while the younger generation may be accustomed to daily showering. People like their baths to be either quick and refreshing or long and hot. Some like to follow this bath with a vigorous rub down with a towel, others will prefer a gentler routine with talcum powder or creams. Wherever possible people should be offered baths at the beginning or the end of the day, to save unnecessary dressing and undressing. Anyone who has been incontinent overnight should be offered a bath or shower. Bath times can be a time for closeness and intimacy and wherever possible assistance with bathing should be provided by the key worker or primary nurse, who should also take responsibility for ensuring that personalised toiletries are always available.

Where people are living at home support should be offered in such a way that the person's routine is disturbed as little as possible. In some cases the facilities in people's own homes will not permit safe bathing and they may be offered a bath as part of a day care programme. Day centre staff can still take account of each person's preferences and ensure that the process is not rushed.

MEALTIMES

People of all classes and cultures place high value on mealtimes. Anyone who has spent a long period of time in an institution will report how food and the occasion of mealtimes become the focus of the day. It is important for staff to ensure that people eat a balanced appetising meal at times that suit them. Good practice dictates that people have a choice of meal, perhaps using photographs of the options as clues (Williams 1990). The meal should be presented in serving dishes wherever possible. If meals have to be pre-plated the staff should take account of people's appetites, likes and dislikes. The crockery and cutlery should be of a normal domestic type, the exception being the provision of specialist dishes for people with a disability. People with dementia should only be given liquidised food on medical direction and medication should never be mixed into food. Whenever possible people should be able to feed themselves, even if this means that they eat mainly 'finger food'. Research has shown that people who are highly dependent have the highest mortality and that elderly people who need to be spoonfed have the worst survival rate of any incapacitated group (Miller 1985). It is possible to organise mealtimes so that people sit at tables for three or four, serve themselves with minimum supervision and where each table has its own condiments, small teapot, milk jug and sugar bowl. There will be accidents and the milk will be poured into the sugar bowl but the benefits outweigh the problems and can be minimised by sympathetic staff intervention. The wearing of bibs and plastic aprons should be minimised, but it is equally inappropriate for people to be wearing food-soiled clothing.

PEOPLE'S POSSESSIONS

In every residential unit there must be a facility for personalising people's own private space, be this a single room or a bed space in a ward. Families should be encouraged to bring in items that are meaningful, the only exception being items of considerable value. Where people have no relatives able to take this role the key worker or primary nurse should be given the time and opportunity to organise this.

Every resident, in every setting, should have access to their own money. Staff need to ensure that money is kept safely and it is not appropriate for people with dementia to have to 'look after' large sums of money. Equally it is not appropriate to refer to personal monies as 'pocket money'. Wherever possible people should be involved in the collection of their pensions and the paying of any bills; the extent of their involvement will have to be determined by their remaining capacity to understand. Many older people with dementia are in a constant state of anxiety because they think bills have not been paid, particularly for their accommodation. It is not helpful for staff to dismiss their anxious queries with a 'don't worry, you don't need to pay anything'. Men should be allowed to carry small change in their trouser pockets and women will be used to having their purse in a handbag. Staff will, inevitably, spend time looking for lost bags and purses but this is a small price to pay for enhancing people's self-esteem.

It appears that staff often underestimate the importance of clothing to a person's self-esteem (Sedgwick 1989). People's clothing should be appropriate to their situation and suitable for the purpose. Cashmere jumpers may be misplaced in long-stay units but the alternative is not necessarily the ubiquitous Crimplene™ dress. Men and women should be encouraged to continue to wear the same type of underwear they have always worn. The stereotype of a bra-less woman with stockings held up by knots is still to be found alongside the man with short trousers with an elasticated waistband. Men's trousers should have flies and be held up by whatever device the person previously wore. A great many accidents are caused by older people with dementia attempting to go to the toilet unaided but finding their clothing unfamiliar. If clothes have to be labelled this should be done discreetly. People should be encouraged to choose what they wear each day but sensitive guidance given so that the end effect is tasteful and in keeping with what is known of their taste in dress (Murphy 1986).

PASSING THE DAY

Once people are up and dressed how do they spend their day? The general public have an impression that the days in units for older people are spent dozing in chairs around the walls. There is an element of truth in this. The chairs may be against the wall to aid staff supervision and minimise the number of things people could trip over and the amount of snoozing may reflect the level of boredom and the over-reliance on medication. Most older people with dementia who live at home do not spend their days in this way and there is no reason why a more normal way of life can not be sustained in every residential unit. The issue of appropriate activities will be dealt with elsewhere in this book but senior staff in each unit should consider whether there are any routines that make normal activity more unlikely.

Are residents able to help lay tables and wash up or are the staff preoccupied with concerns about the additional time this may take and the poor hygiene of some residents? Can the older person launder their own clothes with assistance, dust the furniture or help make scones for tea? Will sufficient staff be on duty to accompany the elderly man who wants to fetch a daily paper from the local shop or pop into the local for a drink? Some readers may think these are unlikely occupations for people with dementia living in an institution but they are more familiar to most older people than colouring in children's painting books or making collages.

RECEIVING VISITORS

Everyone has the right to receive visitors in private; equally, people have the right to choose not to see people who visit. Where people are not accommodated in single rooms there should be a room put aside for visiting. Friends and relatives should be able to visit throughout the day and early evening and should feel able to be involved in the hands-on care of their loved one if they so choose.

Where people are admitted for respite carers are often encouraged, for understandable reasons, to stay away and not visit, in order that they may have a complete rest. Staff need to be aware that this may not be the choice of some relatives who may find that the best recipe for successful respite is where they are relieved of the physical burden of caring but are free to spend time with their relative.

There will be situations where it is appropriate for relatives to stay overnight; care professionals will be accustomed to this at times of serious illness and when people are dying. Thought should be given to making overnight stays a possibility in the early days of admission, when the carer may need reassurance that the staff can provide the right care and the person with dementia would welcome a familiar face. During such a stay the carer can 'teach' the staff the person's routine and preferences and care staff can allay anxieties about the nature of the unit.

BEING A VISITOR IN SOMEONE'S HOME

No matter how demented someone is who lives at home, they must be afforded the respect due to them. Community staff should always introduce themselves on each visit and show an identity card, even if not asked to. They should ask permission before undertaking tasks and should involve the person with all decisions to whatever extent is possible. Apart from ensuring that basic hygiene standards are achieved and maintained care professionals should not try to enforce their standards of cleanliness.

There will be many situations where care professionals are supporting someone with dementia who lives in a house that has many faults and shortcomings; no hot water, trailing flexes, worn carpets and infestations. Those people who manage community-based staff have a responsibility to their staff to ensure that their working conditions are not hazardous or present unacceptable risks. This may mean, on occasions, that a service has to be suspended while problems are resolved: for example, while a house is fumigated. The temporary distress to the householder will have to be balanced against their desire to remain at home for as long as possible.

Many older people with dementia living in the community are supported by their neighbours and local community. Even in those situations where help is not directly provided by neighbours the person's chances of remaining at home may well depend on the tolerance and acceptance of those in the immediate vicinity. This means that community staff must ensure that neighbours and friends are kept informed and involved in care planning, but must balance this against the need to maintain the client's confidentiality. Care professionals should ensure that these issues are regularly discussed in supervision and that individual problems have individual resolutions.

ADMISSION AND DISCHARGE

The welcome that people receive during the first few minutes following arrival may colour their views of the unit permanently. Imagine that you are a carer looking for a unit that will offer respite care for a loved one. Picture three residential units: in the first the doorbell is answered by a neatly dressed member of staff who seems to be expecting you. She takes you to the manager's office and on the way she introduces you to an elderly man who is sitting looking out of the window. In the second unit it takes someone at least 5 minutes to answer the door and a further 2 minutes to undo the locks. They look harassed and surprised to see you. They leave you sitting in the entrance lobby while they find someone you can talk to. They ignore the request for help of a resident sitting by the door. When you visit the third unit the doors are unlocked and open. You walk in and look for a member of staff. No one is in sight but another visitor tells you that she thinks the staff are in the kitchen. You wander around the unit and when you eventually find a staff member they tell you to just wander round and look anywhere you want to. Which unit has convinced you that it has a professional and caring approach?

At the point of admission the new resident should be given time to settle in and time to say their goodbyes. Family members may need time with a member of staff to discuss both practical and emotional issues. Staff will need to make a judgement about how much information a person can absorb during the first few hours and whether or not they can be, or would prefer to be, left alone for a time. Any unit having frequent admissions or offering respite care should expect admissions to take time and occupy individual staff for considerable lengths of time. It makes sense, wherever possible, to try to space out admissions over the week so that each person can be introduced to the unit properly (Gwyther 1985).

Discharges, like admissions, are labour-intensive. There are the practical issues to be dealt with, such as ensuring that all the person's laundry is ready for them and that any medication is prepared for them to take away. The emotional needs of both the resident and the family should be taken into account and the discharge timed for that part of the day when the person with dementia is at their best. Staff should ensure that a person's belongings are sent home with them in a good condition; many carers will infer that the unit that loses glasses or dentures or shrinks knitwear may also have poor practice in personal care.

Where the person was admitted for a period of respite the unit's staff must ensure that any support services previously involved are informed in good time about the discharge. Many units will find it helpful to draw up a simple checklist to ensure that all the tasks associated with discharge have been undertaken. As part of the Community Care Act all Health Authorities have to have agreed discharge policies and all staff in nursing units should be aware of these arrangements. The responsibility for completing the checklist should lie with the primary nurse or key worker.

SEEING THE DOCTOR

In many residential nursing situations and day hospitals the routine of the units seems to revolve around 'seeing the doctor'. There are still units where a weekly ward round is held and patients are expected to talk to a senior doctor about their problems, worries and fears in a public arena. The meeting may be held in a curtained-off part of the ward, allowing other patients to overhear and there may be many people present at the meeting, some of whom have no involvement in the person's care. The power of the medical profession is such, and the ritual so ingrained, that few patients complain. Multidisciplinary working is essential in the care of people with dementia and all members of the team need accurate and up to date information, but there are other ways of ensuring that this happens. Consideration should be given to a scheme where the doctor interviews the patient in private with only the key worker or primary nurse present. A subsequent staff-only meeting can then discuss the information collected and amend the care plan.

In all types of unit people must be given the right to see their doctor alone if they wish and there should be a private space for interviews and examinations.

DEATH AND DYING

There are more rituals associated with death than any other part of institutional life. Some of the rituals will have been developed as a way of sanitising death and minimising the distress caused to staff. Each unit and professional group will have its coded language to describe dying and will have developed policies and procedures to cope with all aspects of death. There will be a defined exit route for the removal of the body, usually by the back door; there will be a ritual associated with clearing and cleaning out the room or bed space of a dead resident and there will be defined and formalised ways of informing (or not) the remaining residents. To care appropriately for someone who is dying is one of the most challenging aspects of caring. The task is neither easier nor less important if the dying person has dementia. The needs of each person as death approaches are different. The needs of their carers vary and the only way of providing good terminal care is by the use of a carefully formulated individual care plan.

ACTION FOR CHANGE

1. Make a note of your routine for baths, speak to the people on your unit and their relatives about their routine at home. Alter your routine to be more appropriate.

2. The primary role of the night staff is to care for the residents. Review the tasks the night staff are regularly asked to undertake and analyse the rationale behind the routine.

3. Undertake an analysis of individual staff's activities over a 2-day period. Use the results to help you identify the method by which work is allocated. Is it the method you thought you were using?

4. List those people in your unit who are on 'soft' diets or being fed liquidised food. Do you know why they can not eat 'normal' food? Involve the community dietitian to assist you in reviewing the practice.

5. Do you have visiting times? Why? How easy is it for a carer to stay for a meal with their relative?

6. How did you come to the conclusion that the residents need to go to the toilet at the time you take them? Review your practice and discuss your assessment methods with your continence adviser.

7. Look at your diary or work schedule for last week. How many appointments did you make on time? You will be aware how distressing it can be for people at home to be uncertain of when help will arrive. What can you do to ensure that your arrival is more predictable?

8. Reflect on the last deaths you have been involved with. Note their similarities and differences. Review your practice; does it ensure that people's religious and cultural practices are honoured? Consider ways of ensuring that staff who have been close to the person who has died have the opportunity to express their feelings.

REFERENCES

Black F (1992) *Primary Nursing. An Introductory Guide.* London: King's Fund Centre.

Gaze H (1990) A good night's Crest. *Nursing Times* **86**(5): 16–17.

Gwyther L (1985) *Care of Alzheimer's Patients: A Manual for Nursing Home Staff.* Washington, DC: AHCA.

Irwin P (1992) Assessing the Individual at Night. In: McMahon R (ed.). *Nursing at Night.* London: Scutari Press.

Kelley L and Lakin J (1988) Role supplementation as a nursing intervention in Alzheimer's disease. *Public Health Nursing* **5**(3): 146–52.

Kron T (1976) *The Management of Patient Care.* Philadelphia: W B Saunders.

Lumley J, Craven J and Aitken J (1980) *Essential Anatomy*, 3rd edn. London: Churchill Livingstone.

Miller A (1985) Nurse/patient dependency – Is it iatrogenic? *Journal of Advanced Nursing* **10**: 63–69.

Murphy E (1986) *Dementia and Mental Illness in the Old.* London: Papermac.

Pearson A (1988) *Primary Nursing.* New York: Croom Helm.

Sedgwick J (1989) Time for a change. *Nursing Times* **85**(48).

Seymour R and Bayer A (1993) Losing track of time: Patient access to clocks and watches. *Care of the Elderly 1993* **5**(6): 240–41.

Totterdell P, Smith L and Folkard S (1992) Nurses as Night Workers. In: McMahon R (ed.). *Nursing at Night.* London: Scutari Press.

Walsh M and Ford P (1989) *Nursing Rituals.* London: Butterworth Heinemann.

Williams W (1990) A photo opportunity. *Nursing Times* **86**(9).

Wright S (1990) *My Patient, My Nurse.* London: Scutari Press.

6 Appropriate Activity
Improving the quality of life through therapeutic interventions

It is clearly acknowledged that dementia can affect anybody. Neither social class nor professional status is a protection against the damage the disease can cause. This knowledge, however, often appears to be ignored when professional care staff are considering how an older person with dementia spends their day, or when they are considering the type of therapeutic interventions that are going to be made available.

How many older people are inflicted with the 'irritation' of being encouraged to play bingo, make wicker baskets or participate in 'singalongs', when they have spent their earlier life running their own business and going to the opera?

It is important to examine the appropriateness of activity. Care professionals should concentrate on providing a wide variety of structured activities that have the potential to provide both 'therapy' and pleasure for older people. Staff need to look positively at what older people with dementia can still achieve and to discover what impaired people can enjoy, within their capabilities and their own social setting. All older people with dementia should be involved in meaningful activity for a part of each day; their level of concentration and involvement will vary but the statement 'they are too demented to do anything' is never appropriate.

The other large area of concern expressed by care professionals is that they do not have time for the 'niceties' of therapy. The authors believe that it is possible to show, in every unit, that appropriate therapies can both preserve older people's skills and reduce 'problem' behaviour, making it a cost-effective intervention.

This chapter considers therapies that are appropriate for people with dementia and will also look at the positive way they can be introduced into a unit or into someone's own home.

POINTS TO PONDER

- Have you visited a friend's house for a drink and been encouraged to join in a game of pontoon, when you really hate playing cards?

- Think of the last time you went into a pub: the juke box was playing loud heavy metal music, when your preference is Beatles' music. Did it spoil your evening?

- Imagine how it must be for somebody who has enjoyed listening to *The Archers* every evening for the past 20 years and then no longer has access to a personal radio.

- Ask staff how comfortable and confident they feel helping out with your current activity programme. How easy do they find it to involve older people?

- List the 'therapies' available to people in your unit. How did you choose them and how long is it since you reviewed their relevance?

- Watch one or two residents throughout the day; for how much time are they involved in activity with other people?

- Reflect on the systems and routines in your unit. Do they help or hinder someone being involved in 'normal' domestic activity (cleaning, cooking, washing up)?

- Think about how you spend your leisure time, list all the activities, highlighting those that you expect to be able to do when you are 70.

WHAT IS NORMAL ACTIVITY?

Before any discussion of therapeutic or diversional activity can take place it is important to think about what can be considered as 'normal activity' for able-bodied, independent people as they age.

The word 'activity' means 'an exertion of energy'. This could be the normal routine of everyday life, repainting the bathroom or the daily walk with the dog. Consider for a moment what may constitute normal activity for an ordinary middle-aged couple.

Betty is 55 and works part time in a department store in the china department. She has been married to Ron for 26 years. They have two grown-up sons, neither of whom is married. Betty does all the food shopping and the housework; she also does the cooking but does not enjoy it. Ron is a retired teacher, who used to referee football matches regularly. He is now on the examiners' board and his hobbies include watching football, playing cards with his wife and tending his allotment.

Betty also enjoys cards and plays Short Mat Bowls, she is the chair of the local village hall committee and serves on the Parish Council. She is a committed Christian, attending church every week. This description, could, with minor changes, fit many couples of a similar age in the United Kingdom.

Consider what would happen if one of them were to develop a dementing illness in the future. Much of their 'normal activity' would be seen as preservable if they were supported at home with community services, but may present some problems in an institutional setting where care staff would have to balance the needs and preferences of Betty and Ron against those of other residents.

People develop their own pattern of therapeutic activity over the course of their life. Even the routines of everyday life are approached differently: someone may do the ironing while drinking a vodka and tonic, others may listen to Vivaldi. It is imperative that care professionals ensure that they know as much about their client as possible. The correct identification of an idiosyncratic activity may mean the difference between a contented person and one who is agitated for 'no apparent reason'.

Older people living in their own homes can choose whether or not they participate in activity, either passive or active, when they have a nap and when they go to bed. These patterns and choices are important to us all and should still exist for people who have dementia and who live in residential settings.

People with dementia are not simply looking for entertainment; they have very special needs and are vulnerable from over-zealous or under-active care professionals who may either herd people into a room to 'do RO' (reality orientation) or, at the other extreme, leave them sitting around the walls becoming isolated and disengaged. The art is to find a balance between the needs of the older person and the resources available. In this context, resources will include staff skills, time and space available.

To understand and accept the need for useful, appropriate activity for people with dementia is as important to their well-being as an appreciation of the need for any practical physical interventions. The managers of a service need to develop a positive approach to activity-based 'therapies' that will assist the staff to find the time and master the skills in order that they can meet the needs of the older person in this arena.

WHY DO ACTIVITIES?

Before considering what activities are appropriate, it is useful to revise why they should be undertaken. As people age there is, usually, a decline in the ability and desire of the person to participate in the more active of pastimes. Older people may not always want to be busy, the quality of the activity being far more important than the duration. The measure of 'successful' activity programmes in institutional settings has often been the amount of activity and the rate of engagement rather than the quality or appropriateness of the activity. Careful consideration needs to be given to the quality and timing of activities. Older people may become exhausted and distressed if they are constantly cajoled into games, craft work or playing bingo with a group of people they barely know. Activity should always be a therapeutic intervention that brings pleasure to the person in a way that they can appreciate. There will be situations where specific therapeutic activity will be 'prescribed' because of the value it may have to the older person, but it is important that this activity should still be in keeping with the person's social and intellectual abilities.

Adapting the environment to meet the needs of the client has already been discussed as a method of coping with someone's antisocial behaviour (Miller 1977). Staff need to be aware that there is a real danger that people with dementia in institutional settings may suffer from sensory deprivation. They may receive restricted stimulation from an austere environment; there may be limited visual stimulation and sparse contact with others (Hallberg, Norberg and Eriksson 1990). In addition there may be few opportunities for conversation with staff and restricted physical stimulation.

There is a proclivity in any care setting for people with dementia to be offered a service that is dominated by physical care with any activity offered having to revolve around the older people's biological needs. People with dementia are often seated in a large room with others but their dementia may be advanced to a stage that does not enable them to interact with the others in the group. People in this situation then appear idle, purposeless and disengaged; silence will be filled with noises of people shouting and the lack of physical activity may result in people wandering and filling their time with their own 'aimless' activities. The usual excuse for this will be that 'there are insufficient staff to do activities and it is not the care professional's job, anyway'. This response cannot be supported. It is the care professional's job to involve themselves in activity, not only because it is cost-effective, reducing people's disruptive behaviour (Smith-Jones and Francis 1992) but also because it forms an essential part of an individualised care package. Staff can not claim to take a 'holistic perspective' if they disregard this aspect of normal life.

To offer activity that fosters dignity, personal identity and improves self-esteem can be shown to improve people's behaviour and give them a more settled night (Smith-Jones and Francis 1992). The impact of an effective activity programme can be measured in less 'problem behaviour' and the need for less medication.

FOSTERING DEPENDENCE – DO CARE PROFESSIONALS REINFORCE THE PROBLEMS?

Up to 80 per cent of interactions in a residential setting will be related to physical care, with most 'conversations' with clients being restricted to informing or questioning, leaving little room for relationship formation (Salmon 1993). It is easy to assume that if care professionals have a positive attitude towards older people they will automatically engage in providing more activity. This is not confirmed and it is more likely that there is virtually no positive correlation between a nurse's attitudes and their enthusiasm to involve older people in activity.

A positive attitude towards older people should encompass the empowering of clients and the encouragement of independence and choice. Perhaps within the caring professions the 'all doing – all caring' approach is still considered as a positive attribute. This in itself can often be damaging; if clients are allowed to take less responsibility for their own lives, they inevitably become more dependent on others. If the care professional takes over the lead role in all decision-making or in all personal care, the older person will respond by showing reduced activity and lowered morale (Eddington et al 1990). If a person feels that they are not allowed to take responsibility for themselves it is likely that they will also feel a degree of dissatisfaction with life. The research of Eddington et al (1990) involved older people who were articulate and who could be used as a comparative reflection of the views of older people with dementia, who may not be able to articulate their frustrations and anxieties about being in an institutional care setting, or of being dependent on community support services. Encouraging dependence, however well intentioned and however unconsciously conducted, will only devalue the person's self-worth and increase, in the long term, the care professional's workload.

All humans will strive to maximise the control they have over their lives. There is a challenge for institutions to find ways to acknowledge this. All too often, at the end of a long line of bureaucratic processes will be the older person who is dementing, and who is rarely involved in the decision-making processes. It is vital that care professionals find ways of helping older people retain their independence and of reinforcing the benefit of independence. Many traditional care settings have routines and rituals that reinforce dependence and helplessness. Learned helplessness may occur when a person is attempting to control a situation: for instance, an older person who has been ill and dependent on a relative may see that they would lose their relative's attention and sympathy if they got well, so they choose to continue to require assistance. Similarly, within an institution a person may see that there are benefits and rewards associated with certain behaviours (Robertson 1986).

It is important that staff show respect to the older person and are appropriately generous with praise. Staff must assume that all older people with dementia can hear and understand comments made by staff and that adverse comments may affect their self-esteem. Staff should also encourage and ensure that even the most impaired clients are 'allowed' to be involved in the simplest of activities, perhaps watering the plants. Encouraging involvement leads to an increase in alertness and a consequent improvement in quality of life (Robertson 1986).

There are, of course, a range of therapeutic reasons for people to participate in activity; those with dementia need to remain physically active to prevent stiffness, muscle spasm and wasting. Activity can prevent a reduction in cardiac output and help with a disturbed sleep/wake pattern. Physical and psychological activities will assist the older person to remain at their potential and encourage them to feel valued, motivated and have a sense of dignity within their disease. These positive attributes will be reflected in the client's calmer inner self and will, in turn, reduce the management requirements caused by their disease. The care professional has a duty of care to the older person in their care and this duty of care must include the prevention of problems. Take the example of an older person who, while living at home, was able to carry out a range of normal domestic tasks that kept her ambulant, active, involved and in control. If this person becomes confused and enters a care setting they may suffer from a range of problems associated with their inability to initiate these domestic tasks. These can be illustrated diagrammatically, as shown below.

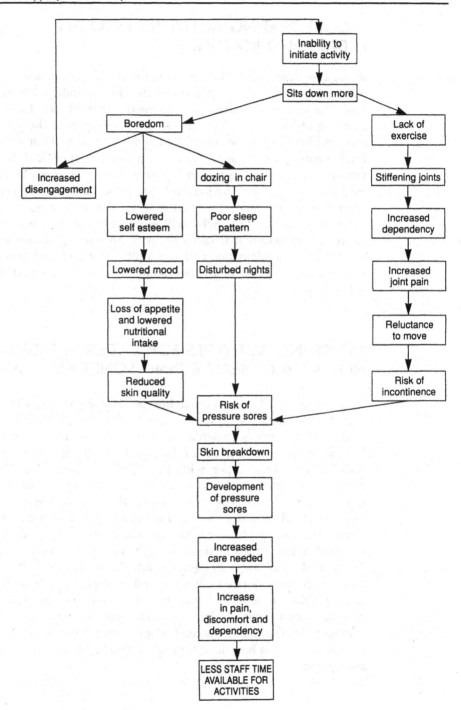

INCORPORATING ACTIVITIES INTO AN ESTABLISHED ROUTINE

If person-centred activities are not already a part of the ethos of the residential setting it is important to develop a strategy for implementation. The aim of this strategy is to ensure that all staff have an understanding about why activity needs to become part of the philosophy of care and how it will be introduced. The fundamental cornerstone when implementing this change, in a regimented routine that is geared to physical care, is for the project leader to have a clear vision about what they want to achieve. The person leading the change must have a strong commitment and believe in what they are doing; they must also be able to identify the key staff who will support the change within the unit. There are numerous management styles and an equal number of ways of implementing activities within a unit; a method that was successful in one may not be so in another. Some key points may usefully be considered.

IMPROVING ACTIVITIES FOR OLDER PEOPLE MAY NOT ALWAYS MEAN DOING SOMETHING NEW

There may already be 'normal life' activity going on within the unit that staff can incorporate into a person's day. The staff need to be aware of the older person's preferences; some may be able and may wish to help with the washing up or laying of the tables. Some may enjoy assisting the housekeeper with the dusting, others may like nothing better than watching the Test Match or listening to *The Archers*. The key to successful activity is to ensure that the person who wants to listen to *The Archers* does not end up watching the Test Match! In other words, the care professional should know their clients well. It is not sufficient to know their medical or social history. The person with dementia has had a full life with agonies and pleasures, jobs and hobbies, and these experiences can be built upon and used positively. The information can be obtained either informally while chatting, through formal or informal reminiscence, or by a conscious proactive approach. This latter approach is the most successful and systematic way of obtaining information and is best done through a structured social and recreational assessment.

IMPLEMENTING EXTRA ACTIVITIES

If staff are keen to offer the clients a positive experience and work towards maintaining independence, self-esteem and dignity, it may well involve more than simply 'normal life activity'. Time may need to be found to incorporate some structured activity. This can be achieved by looking carefully at time management within the unit and re-examining the priority given to different tasks. On even the busiest of units it should be possible to identify a time slot of 15 minutes that could be set aside for an appropriate intervention. It may be, perhaps, a physical activity to stimulate and improve people's circulation. Once one or two keen members of staff have shown what can be achieved and how much some older people can enjoy a physical activity, it can encourage the more sceptical staff, and more slots of time may suddenly become visible. For many personal therapeutic interventions usually only short periods of time are required but they must be regularly available; for someone with severe dementia it may be appropriate to spend 10 minutes a day with them, holding their hand and chatting to them (as one would do if they were able to respond). This activity would need to be included in the person's care plan and given priority within the routine of the day, giving it equal status with tasks associated with physical care.

ACTIVITY FOR ACTIVITY'S SAKE

Two stereotypical views of staff relate to activity. First, 'we were told to do some activities so that's what we are doing. All our 24 residents will do bingo on Mondays, craft on Tuesday, singalongs on Thursdays, and make fluffy balls on Fridays'; or, secondly, where staff have failed, or never tried to implement activities, 'our residents don't like doing things, they're too old to be busy, they like dozing in the chair.'

Other horrific scenarios will have been experienced by most care professionals; establishments where the TV is switched on at 9 a.m. and flashes pictures constantly in the corner of the room, while a pop music station on the radio blasts out simultaneously in the other corner; or groups of older people watching staff make collages from discarded birthday cards to be put on the wall to make a monthly calendar.

These negative degrading scenarios are all too frequent within all types of residential setting and have no place in high quality care. The value of activity has already been established; it is important, however, to ensure that it is as near as possible 'tailor-made' for each individual.

REGIMENTATION VERSUS SPONTANEITY

If the unit is fortunate enough to have a music therapist, for example, the rationale for the group session should be clearly identified and people encouraged to go if it meets their needs. There will be little or no value in running an hour-long session for all the people on the unit, levelling the session at the abilities of the least-able person. The result will be that those who are more able will only become demoralised or bored. Alternatively, if the session is aimed at the most competent, there will be participants who became discouraged and who may have their inabilities emphasised. Two small groups tailored to meet different needs must be preferable and more productive; the planning of any activity must include the identification of the benefits of the specific activity and an assessment of how well it will meet the needs and match the desires of specific clients. Some care professionals feel that there should be no planning and all activities should be spontaneous, depending both on how the clients feel and on the workload of the unit. This is a naive approach to the provision of activities. Planning is vital if staff who have a specific interest and skill in a particular therapy are to organise the resources for the group and make themselves available. In normal life most things have an element of planning. When visiting the dentist an appointment needs to be made, with a compromise on the most suitable time. When going to see an artist in concert no compromise is possible: one either sees the show at the time advertised or misses the event. However, going for an afternoon stroll may well be dictated by the weather; thus normal life has large elements of structure, routine and organisation interspersed by occasional spontaneous activity and for people with dementia it should be no different.

Having an outline plan of when things should occur will help with practical aspects of organising activity, but it should not be treated with rigidity. As clients are forgetful they may find it useful to be given a card or simple diary sheet to remind them of what they could be involved with, if they wish. Again, in everyday life, able-bodied people are not expected to remember all of their appointments; by knowing in advance, people can plan their day and this aspect should not be overlooked just because people have dementia. It has to be acknowledged that for some older people an appointment card may cause some anxiety. The appropriateness of this system will need to be judged on an individual basis.

USING STAFF PRODUCTIVELY

Not every care professional will be able to be involved in all types of activity. It is important that a good leader identifies what qualities each staff member has and what specific skills they can bring to enhance the life of the client. Obvious therapeutic skills of specialists should be acknowledged and used to the benefit of the clients.

Once a small amount of activity is successfully implemented in a unit in a non-threatening way, care professionals who previously had little interest may enjoy the interaction; for example, staff may see the benefit of offering clients the option to undertake gentle exercise or 'keep fit' and as a result may be keen to pursue Extend training (Copple 1987). The activity chosen as the first 'trial' activity should be carefully selected; it must be 'failure free' for staff and residents and should be led by an enthusiastic and confident staff member. Remember, nothing succeeds like success!

Many acknowledged therapies can be introduced into a unit following appropriate training and courses are usually accessible through professional development departments. It is, however, just as important to utilise the expertise that the care professional has from their own social lifestyle. A member of staff may, in their spare time, enjoy carpentry, fishing or candlelight suppers! Any of these may be appropriate to specific clients and can help relationships develop from a basis of mutual respect and understanding. It is also important to acknowledge the specific skills required to facilitate specific activities and so it may be necessary to withdraw a specific activity if a member of staff is away, rather than appear to trivialise the value of what they do by simply handing it over to somebody else.

For staff who are involved in the more essential aspects of care, being responsible for a specific therapeutic intervention in which they have an interest can encourage them and improve their feelings of self-worth and increase their job satisfaction. Specific training can offer unqualified staff certain practical skills, thus making them a specialist within the team. Examples of these could include manicure, hairdressing, aromatherapy, reflexology or massage.

MOTIVATING 'UNWILLING' CLIENTS

To a certain extent people's level of motivation and involvement is part of their character and in every residential setting there will be a few who will be self-motivating. Motivation is not a tangible commodity. It can be affected by many factors: emotional and physical health, time, place and the company one is a part of all play a part (Armstrong 1987). It has been said that there is little 'therapeutic' difference between enforced activity and enforced inactivity and the difference between encouraging participation and enforcing participation is just as fine. It is important, therefore, that care professionals are able to read and interpret the client's body language; sometimes people say 'no' and mean 'no'. Sometimes the message may be 'well, I'd like to but I don't want to burden you', or it may mean 'no, I think I'm supposed to be doing something else', or 'I'd love to but I can't afford it'. The art is to judge the response and encourage accordingly, deciphering what the older person really means by 'no'. Only the care professional who knows the client well can determine how much pressure to put on a specific client as this, used inappropriately, could damage the value of the activity and cause distress. However, it is not always appropriate to accept the first refusal and encouragement may in the end be fruitful. Gore (1993) suggests that the key words are ability, readiness and opportunity. If these three factors are acknowledged, success should follow.

ACTIVITIES AND THERAPIES – WHAT SHOULD BE DONE

Throughout this chapter the term 'activity' has been used to mean every type of intervention that a care professional undertakes, which cannot be classified as physical care. The term does not adequately reflect the individual-sensitive approach to activity that is so often required by people with dementia. The term 'personal therapeutic intervention' (PTI) provides a more accurate description of the types and purposes of activity and so will be used in preference. Personal therapeutic interventions for people with dementia have to have one factor above all others, that they are failure-free and that they bring moment to moment satisfaction for the person with dementia. The person may not remember exactly what it was that made them feel happy but they will continue to be aware of their feeling of self-worth or satisfaction (Sheridan 1992). It is pertinent to review different types of activity and discuss their relevance to people with dementia. Some traditional activities, e.g. bingo, were found to be unsuccessful in some day centres because of the fine language and motor skills required (Sheridan 1992), yet this is one activity in which care professionals may unwittingly engage clients, thinking that it is both easy and undemanding. When look-ing at any therapeutic intervention it is important to know why it is being considered; running a reality orientation group because it impresses the manager is not a good enough reason.

NORMAL LIFE ACTIVITY AS A THERAPY

A therapeutic activity for one person may be quite boring and irrelevant to another. Normal life therapy is probably the most individual therapy of all, as it seeks to replicate parts of the person's premorbid life, utilising the skills that they have learned from the past. This enables the person to be in control, as they are the knowledgeable 'expert' in the subject. This in turn raises their self-esteem and makes them feel valued. There is a danger that being asked to take part in therapeutic interventions that are based on activities from the past may confirm to the person that they are not as able as they were to undertake these tasks. Normal life therapy can include taking the person to the shops to do their own shopping, going with the care professional in the car to collect their prescription, having their hair done or watching their favourite TV programme. The care professional should also consider that periods of inactivity are important; someone may wish to sit and do nothing or spend the afternoon lying on their bed. Many people have, throughout their lives, developed a preference for the way they rest during the day. Some may doze after lunch in a chair, others may choose to lie on the bed, if they have the chance, and this should be considered a therapeutic intervention. The skill is to encourage the person to balance periods of rest and activity, as both are as important as each other.

Activity should be seen as important no matter how disabled or confused a person is. Even people who are severely damaged by the disease process may still gain pleasure from simple day to day activity; having someone sit and chat to them, reading a newspaper article to them or just sitting alongside them all show the older person that they are important and valued simply for being themselves.

In some residential settings older people are encouraged to participate in helping with the washing up or table laying. In others it is emphatically resisted because of hygiene. An element of moderation is needed. Not every client presents a health hazard and these simple tasks may help the person feel valued. Where people are still living at home they should be encouraged to continue with any household tasks that they are used to undertaking. They should also be encouraged to keep in touch with their friends, families and local community. Both at home and in a residential setting, there are gains for both the older person and their family if they can be kept in touch and assisted to mark birthdays or anniversaries in the family by helping them in the purchase and sending of cards and presents.

The most important aspects of normal life therapy are to raise the person's self-esteem, their feelings of self-worth and awareness or reality by allowing them to be themselves. To find out what 'makes each resident tick' and then utilising it will reduce many other management problems and make the person feel good about themselves (Armstrong 1987).

As discussed in other chapters the milieu of a residential setting is an integral part of someone's care. This must, of course, include the atmosphere created by the type of conversation and light-hearted but respectful approach taken by staff. In the USA this, not surprisingly perhaps, has been taken one step further and Humour Therapy is becoming a recognised treatment for many patients with a range of conditions. It has been found to be physiologically beneficial, improving ventilation, increasing blood oxygen and circulation, stimulating the person to produce their own painkillers and waking people up who are normally drowsy (Carlisle 1990). Hospitals in the USA are even employing 'humour nurses' to encourage positive laughter. It is felt to be uplifting, diverts people from feeling self-pity; it relieves anxiety and breaks the cycle of stress (Pasquali 1990). The benefits can easily be imagined, as individuals who feel happy can have a dramatic affect on the atmosphere and therefore other people in a shared environment. It should only be considered, however, within normal activity and with due consideration of the person's cultural and social status.

USING THERAPIES

A range of therapies are perceived to be particularly relevant to people with dementia, for example Reminiscence, Reality Orientation and Occupational Therapy. Others are less often considered to be appropriate to use, such as art therapy, music therapy or complementary therapies. If one believes that no two people with dementia are alike, and that people with dementia should be treated as individuals, then it becomes clear that it is not helpful to consider some activities and therapies as suitable for people with dementia and others as unsuitable.

It has been recognised by psychologists that they have tended to leave others to undertake psychological therapies, and that the direct involvement of psychologists as clinicians with people with dementia has been rather limited (Hanley and Gilhooly 1986). They feel that this has meant that some 'therapies' have been undertaken by well intentioned but poorly trained care professionals and many of the psychological benefits of the intervention have been lost. It needs to be debated, therefore, if there is fundamentally any difference between activities that are carried out for very specific reasons and therapies. The use of the word therapy has a more professional air about it and yet if the psychologists are correct in their assumptions the interventions have no more value than activities conducted for diversional reasons.

It is argued by the authors that both interventions need to be conducted by care professionals who have been trained to undertake and understand the rationale for the intervention. On this assumption both activities and therapies are of equal importance, provided they are used appropriately.

SOME EXAMPLES OF THERAPIES

Reality Orientation (RO)

Reality Orientation (RO) was first developed in the USA in 1958; since then it has spread throughout the world. There are three major types of RO; basic RO or 24-hour RO, RO classes and advanced RO. Twenty-four-hour RO is a continual process whereby staff present information reminding the person constantly of the time and place, confused speech is not reinforced and there are always large, rather institutional signs to tell people where they are. RO classes involve a small group of older people and a member of staff meeting regularly for a structured session. They are usually held to support 24-hour RO but may be done in isolation. The third type, advanced RO, is where wide-ranging topics are discussed (Holden and Woods 1982). The problem, however, is that often people with dementia are lumped together and their different psychological deficits are not considered. Formal qualification is not considered necessary to practise RO (Holden and Woods 1982). Enthusiasm alone is felt to be the only necessary qualification, but it is a therapeutic intervention that does need to be practised and delivered with great skill. There is also limited evidence on the long-term effects of RO (Hanley 1986), but it is acknowledged that, provided the staff continue to follow a positive approach throughout the day, RO can be useful and cost-effective (Hanley 1986).

Reminiscence Therapy

Reminiscence therapy is completely different from RO. It has the key aim of using people's life experiences to highlight the older person's remaining skills and abilities, rather than highlighting their deficits. Everyone reminisces. It is normal activity for people of any age and is usually perceived as enjoyable. Using reminiscence as a therapeutic intervention has become popular but staff must be aware that in some situations it can have negative effects.

There are three main ways that reminiscence therapy can be used; first, as a social tool in a large group, perhaps as a singalong, or the watching of a film; secondly, on an individual basis to help develop relationships and improve interpersonal communication, and thirdly, as a group activity to improve communication skills, raise self-esteem and channel ruminating thought patterns (O'Donovan 1993). Reminiscence therapy is not a history lesson. It is irrelevant to the outcome of the session whether or not the information discussed is chronologically correct. The session should encourage the client to be the person who is in control: they have the knowledge and the experience and the care professional should not be didactic in their approach. Some people do not like to reminisce and for them involvement in such activity will be detrimental (Coleman 1988); for example, not everyone will have pleasant memories of the war and want to talk about it. It is again a therapeutic intervention that should not be undertaken lightly. The aim of its introduction should be clearly identified. The main benefits for the staff must be a better understanding of the client and their life; the benefit for the older person should be a feeling of a positive energy that leaves them content and at peace.

The therapeutic value of reminiscence when used with people with dementia is in doubt; there is not sufficient evidence to support the hypothesis that confused people experience any cognitive or behavioural changes as a result of reminiscing and, at best, it is perhaps seen as an enjoyable diversional pastime (Thornton and Brotchie 1987). Anecdotal evidence shows, however, that if older people are given the opportunity to use their life experience in a positive way it can raise their self-esteem and make them feel valued (Phair and Elsey 1990).

Validation Therapy

For 20 years Naomi Feil has been developing a unique approach to communicating with elderly disorientated people. The method is based on the theory that very old people struggle to resolve unfinished life issues before death. Their behaviour reflects this in four specific progressive stages: malorientation, time confusion, repetitive motion and vegetation. There are, in turn, very specific techniques to help with individuals at each stage (Feil 1992). These techniques include empathy, reminiscing, touch and mirroring. In the latter stages of deterioration objects that are important to the older person may be replaced symbolically by other everyday items, thus the pair of socks that someone constantly plays with may represent a small child. Similarly, movements may represent motherhood and safety. The therapy can either be undertaken individually and informally, or in small groups of six to eight people, the group lasting no longer than 20 minutes. Prompts such as music or photographs can be used in the sessions but only to aid communication with the disorientated person in whatever reality they are, in order to ease distress and restore self-worth (Bleathman and Morton 1988).

Limited studies have been carried out by Naomi Feil to assess the benefits of this therapy (Feil 1989). The research did not include the examination of a control group, and there is little discussion in the research account of how much change was due to the pathological changes of the disease process or the extra attention these people had received.

Validation has been used in a few establishments within the United Kingdom. In one study a group of elderly people participated in a series of 20 group sessions. It was identified that there was a marked contrast between the lack of meaningful interaction observed outside the group and the members' ability to maintain and discuss themes for 5 minutes within the group. The researchers of this study acknowledge, however, that it was not established how much of this improvement was due to the validation therapy and how much was due to the structure of the group and the manufactured environment (Bleathman and Morton 1992).

Music Therapy

Music is much in evidence to hearing people every day, whether live, on record, on the radio or television. Some music will arouse, some subdue and some relax; it is evocative of sensations and emotions, it can affect the mood as it contains both persuasive and suggestive elements (Alvin 1966). The effect it provokes depends on the different elements of sound and their relationship within the tune. The general aim of music therapy when used with people with dementia is to meet the emotional, social and spiritual needs of the clients and thus improve their self-esteem and quality of life. Music therapy can be used for different reasons within a clinical setting and can be beneficial within someone's own home. It can be used by a qualified music therapist to assess memory, general knowledge, to stimulate movement and even rekindle feelings. This should be done with great sensitivity, as music can provoke a range of negative and positive feelings. For those staff who work with people with dementia, specific aims can be worked towards. In a small group music can help to rebuild social bridges, emphasising the person's positive attributes and giving them the opportunity to take control by choosing the music. If the group is small and kept to a limited session music can help reduce aggression and agitation, both by the mood of the music and by the active engagement of the older person.

Music can be used in a therapeutic way by an enthusiast, either professional or voluntary, if approached in a positive social setting. Many older people can recall some parts of songs if they are prompted and many care professionals will have been surprised to see profoundly confused people being able to remember whole songs and appear animated, even for a short while (Brooker 1991). In this way music can help carers to see the person behind the dementia and appreciate their 'personhood'. Cathartic outbursts can occur even if a person has requested a song and the care professional should be available to counsel the person and support the music facilitator at all times.

Other voluntary groups such as the 'Council for Music in Hospitals' will perform concerts large or small in hospitals or care settings for any client group. They see music as a means of communication that has the power to penetrate the innermost human soul, and as such can be invaluable to millions of people in residential care (Lindsay 1993). Music should be a way of creating a positive atmosphere. It will only do this if the music is at an appropriate level and appropriate in nature. In some units personal stereos are provided in order to ensure that each client can listen to whatever they want.

Pet Therapy

For people who live at home having a pet can offer companionship and may both relieve stress and encourage exercise. The 'Pat-a-Dog' service is now operating in many parts of the country and will provide regular visits for appropriately trained dogs. To have a dog in a unit may be very comforting for some and offer a focus for their affections but the consequences of having an animal, particularly a dog, should be considered quite seriously. It will undoubtedly assist in creating a domestic atmosphere and may improve communication and counteract some of the negative consequences of institutionalisation.

One study in Australia, however, found that the perceived benefits of the dog were greater that the actual benefits and, although the dog initially acted as a catalyst for conversation, after 6 months the residents had become used to the animal and the benefits disappeared. The staff, however, remained more enthusiastic about the benefits of the dog than the residents (Winkler et al 1989). This should not dampen people's enthusiasm for having a 'unit pet', but should remind staff of the need to think carefully about the practicalities of having a pet, weighing these against the estimated benefits of an animal.

Using Children to Raise Self-esteem

Interacting with children is a pleasure often denied to older people, particularly as they dement. With the traditional nuclear family no longer the norm, many older people do not see their grandchildren or great-grandchildren as much as they would have done in years gone by. Children, particularly those under school age, are accepting of people and do not see handicaps or disfigurement as an adult would. They are not as judgemental as adults and so can have a very positive effect on the elderly, exhibiting spontaneous engagement and showing positive regard. People who are in the early stages of dementia and who live in the community may benefit from associating with children, perhaps at playgroups (Smith 1990), or by being invited to school plays, assemblies or, if they are still able to, by offering a lap at a day nursery. Older children and those doing community service projects would be valuable within a residential setting to engage the older person by reading or writing letters, or simply befriending (Dopson 1989). Using the valuable resource of children and adolescents can add a new emphasis to the environment and ethos of the unit.

THERAPEUTIC INTERVENTIONS FOR PLEASURE

The list of activities that can be used to bring pleasure to somebody with dementia is endless and many are already in regular use both in the residential setting and the community. The key issue to consider is, however, whether the intervention to be offered is in keeping with the person's lifestyle. The activity must be relevant to the person. There is no point in asking someone to participate in a crossword, however well it is adjusted to their cognitive skills, if they have always loathed them. The intervention should not be patronising: a jigsaw with only 12 pieces, for example, would be appropriate for someone if it had an adult orientated picture on it; but a 12-piece puzzle with a picture of Thomas the Tank Engine would be demeaning and highlight the failing abilities of the older person.

The fundamental principles of any intervention are that it must:

• be simple – but hard enough for the person to feel they have succeeded;
• be appropriate to the premorbid ability of the person;

- offer variety;
- be more than a means of 'killing time';
- focus on the remaining abilities of the person, however restricted they may be; and
- avoid too much choice, as this will cause confusion (Sheridan 1992).

Interventions do not need to be sophisticated or complicated; a trip in a car to do some shopping, or an excursion to the countryside or the accompanying of someone on a car journey to collect something from the town, can often be satisfying for someone who does not often get out. Unit activities, such as tea dances, quizzes, videos or special meals, can help to generate a positive social milieu. These activities should not be restricted to the Christmas period; regular social functions help to raise the morale of staff as well as build relationships with clients and their families.

USING SPECIALISTS AND VOLUNTEERS

Implementing a personal therapeutic intervention programme will only be successful if it encompasses the whole spectrum of specialist services that are available. This discussion has only examined a small proportion of interventions and activities that can be undertaken. Many more are facilitated by specialists, such as art therapy, occupational therapy, speech therapy and complementary therapy and will all have specific contributions to make in improving the quality of life of someone who has dementia. The care professional has the key role of coordinating appropriate interventions and furthering their use within residential settings and the community. Considering the role of volunteers as a source of person-power can ensure that there are enough people around a unit to facilitate activity. There is a particularly important role for volunteers in assisting with those clients whose previous hobbies have taken them out of the home, perhaps to watch football or going for a ramble. These activities are 'labour intensive', requiring one to one staffing. There will be a need to ensure that the volunteer is well vetted, matched to the client and appropriately skilled. Volunteer programmes must always be dealt with seriously with a designated senior member of staff being given the time and the responsibility for organising vetting, training and supervision.

If a group of care professionals can make the transition from traditional, physical, custodial care by reviewing attitudes and approaches and fostering an active stimulating care environment, the effect will not only be encouraging for the older people but will have a domino effect on the staff working in the unit and a more positive overall attitude towards the clients will follow. Seeing clients doing more than simply sitting, seeing them achieve, seeing them respond and seeing them smile will have a profound effect on the staff and raise everyone's morale (Jones 1988).

ACTION FOR CHANGE

1. Undertake an audit of the amount of activity currently provided in your unit: consider asking someone unconnected with your service to do this. They should observe the unit on several occasions for at least half a day each time.

2. Discuss with each staff member what their own hobbies include and what therapeutic activities they would be interested to be involved in.

3. Look at how you collect information about the preferred lifestyle of people being admitted. If your system does not provide the right information, design a more appropriate one.

4. Decide on one activity to implement, either for an individual client or for a group. Identify the member of staff to be involved and the most appropriate time of day to ensure its success. Decide on the equipment that will be needed and have it available in good time.

5. Evaluate any new therapeutic initiative by taking the baseline of the person's physical and mental well-being before the activity and note any changes during and after the intervention.

6. Examine how staff undertaking activities are currently supported. Discuss with them ways of improving the situation.

7. Review the unit's policies and routines to see if the amount of 'normal life activity' that currently occurs could be increased by a change in approach.

8. Examine ways of increasing the amount and range of activities available to people who are supported in their own home; explore what local resources could be utilised. Where appropriate clubs and groups are scarce consider ways of working with other agencies to develop small local schemes.

REFERENCES

Alvin J (1966) *Music Therapy*. London: John Baker Publishers.

Armstrong J (1987) *Staying Active: A Positive Approach in Residential Homes*. London: Centre for Policy on Ageing.

Bleathman C and Morton I (1988) Validation therapy with the demented elderly. *Journal of Advanced Nursing* 13(4): 511–14.

Bleathman C and Morton I (1992) Validation therapy: extracts from 20 groups with dementia sufferers. *Journal of Advanced Nursing* 17: 658–66.

Brooker E (1991) Just a song at twilight. *Nursing Times* 87(38): 32–34.

Carlisle D (1990) Comic relief. *Nursing Times* 86(38): 50–51.

Coleman P (1988) Issues in the therapeutic use of reminiscence with elderly people. *Mental Health Problems in Old Age*. Chichester: John Wiley.

Copple P (1987) Movement is life. *Geriatric Nursing and Home Care* 7(10): 20–22.

Dopson L (1989) The Generation Game. *Nursing Times* 85(50): 32–33.

Eddington C, Piper J, Tanna B, Hodkinson H, and Salmon P (1990) Relationships between happiness, behavioural status and dependency on others in elderly patients. *British Journal of Clinical Psychology* 29: 43–50.

Feil N (1989) *Validation: the Feil Method. How to Help Disoriented Old*. Ohio: Edward Feil Productions.

Feil N (1992) Honesty, the best policy. *Nursing the Elderly* 4(5): 10–12.

Gore I (1993) *Age and Vitality: Common Sense Ways of Adding Life to Your Years*. London: Allen & Unwin.

Halberg I, Norberg A and Eriksson S (1990) A comparison between the care of vocally disruptive patients and that of other residents at Psychogeriatric Wards. *Journal of Advanced Nursing* 15: 410–16.

Hanley I (1986) Reality orientation in the care of the elderly patient with dementia. In: Hanley I and Gilhooly M (eds) *Psychological Therapies for the Elderly*. London: Croom Helm.

Hanley I and Gilhooly M (eds) (1986) *Psychological Therapies for the Elderly*. London: Croom Helm.

Holden V and Woods R (1982) *Reality Orientation: Psychological Approaches to the Confused Elderly*. London: Churchill Livingstone.

Jones R (1988) Experimental study to evaluate nursing staff morale in a high stimulation geriatric psychiatry setting. *Journal of Advanced Nursing* 13: 352–57.

Lindsay S (1993) Musical care. *Nursing Standard* 7(19): 20–21.

Miller E (1977) The management of dementia. A review of some possibilities. *British Journal of Clinical Psychology* 16: 77–83.

O'Donovan S (1993) The memory lingers on. *Elderly Care*. 5(1): 27–31.

Pasquali E (1990) Learning to laugh: humour as therapy. *Journal of Psychological Nursing* 28(3): 31–35.

Phair L and Elsey I (1990) Sharing memories. *Nursing Times* 86(27): 50–52.

Robertson I (1986) Learned helplessness. *Nursing Times* 82(51): 28–30

Salmon P (1993) Interaction of nurses with elderly patients: relationships to nurses' attitudes and to formal activity periods. *Journal of Advanced Nursing* 18(1): 14–19.

Sheridan C (1992) *Failure Free Activities for the Alzheimer's Patient*. London: Macmillan.

Smith J (1990) Feeling useful again. *Nursing Times* 86(27): 48–50.

Smith–Jones S and Francis G (1992) Disruptive institutionalised elderly: a cost effective intervention. *Journal of Psychosocial Nursing* 30(10): 17–20.

Thornton S and Brotchie J (1987) Reminiscence: a critical review of the empirical literature. *British Journal of Clinical Psychology* **26**: 93–111.

Winkler A, Fairnie H, Gericeuich F and Long M (1989) The impact of a resident dog on an institution for the elderly: effects on perceptions and social interactions. *The Gerontologist* **29**(2): 216–23.

7 Carers
Developing partnerships

The word 'carer' was rarely seen or heard before the 1970's. Since then issues relating to carers have been examined widely, partly as a result of the rise of the feminist movement.

Caring for someone can be fulfilling and rewarding or a period of exhaustion and frustration. The experience of caring is unique to each relationship but there are common themes and problems that staff need to be aware of.

Caring is a job with a difference: it has no fixed hours or wages and few tangible rewards. As a carer you are not viewed by the government as being either 'employed' or contributing to the productivity of the nation, yet it has been estimated that carers save the government an estimated £24 billion a year (Kelling 1993). Caring always has an intimate relationship at its core, which can be both its strength and its weakness. Few people see themselves as carers, which may help explain the poor take-up of some services designed and advertised as being for carers and many carers are elderly people looking after equally elderly friends and relatives.

It is vital that professional care staff address seriously the issues that affect carers, that they examine their own attitudes and beliefs about carers and consider ways of improving the service they can offer. In particular it is important to recognise the contribution of carers and the need to work in partnership with them.

POINTS TO PONDER

- How often do you involve carers in care planning, reviews and the formulation of policy?

- Think about a particular carer; do you know where their emotional support comes from? Are you confident that you know what aspect of caring they find most difficult?

- Think about your colleagues. Are you aware if any of them have personal experiences of caring?

- Have you ever involved carers in your training programmes?

- Do you think people are less caring now than in former times?

- Do you assess and record carers' needs?

- Do you feel confident that you and your service are sensitive to the needs of carers from ethnic minority groups?

- How do you collect and collate carers' views about your service?

A PORTRAIT OF CARING

How many carers are there?

If this book had been written 20 years ago there would have probably been no reference to carers. If the book had been written 10 years ago there would have been references to 'formal' and 'informal' carers. The term 'informal carer' was used to denote those people who were not paid to care and was viewed by many people as a derogatory term. The preferred terms now are 'family carer' with 'formal carer' still being occasionally used to describe those people employed in caring agencies.

The growth in awareness of the impact of caring has led to much research and the founding of numerous carers' associations has ensured that carers' issues are kept on the political agenda. In spite of this it is still difficult to establish how many carers there are in the country and in particular, how many carers are looking after people with dementia.

In 1985 the General Household Survey first asked questions that related to caring. When the information was published 3 years later it stated that there were up to 6 million carers in Britain. This is equivalent to 14 per cent of the adult population. (Twigg 1992). Since this date there has been considerable speculation about whether this figure is accurate and what kinds of caring situations are included. Closer examination shows that the 6 million figure included both people who were 'primary carers', that is, people usually living in the same household as the person they cared for, and 'secondary carers' – those who assisted other people to a much lesser degree and who may not live in the same household. A recent reinterpretation of the statistics leads researchers to think that there may be nearer to 1.3 million (i.e. 4 per cent) 'primary carers' in Britain (Parker 1990).

While there may be fewer carers than first thought there is no doubt that the number of hours they give assistance and the range of tasks they undertake is substantial. Obviously, all these figures relate to carers in general, it being difficult to estimate what proportion of caring relationships involve someone with dementia, but one can be confident that the numbers will be substantial.

Who are they?

If one examines the relationship of carers to the person they assist it is clear that spouses are most commonly involved in caring. The next most common relationship would be that of son/daughter and son-in-law/daughter-in-law. It is noteworthy that up to 10 per cent of carers are estimated to be helping support someone who is not related to them at all.

The gender of the carer has an impact on how they perceive the task, how well they may succeed and on how professionals will view them. It is a commonly held view that the vast majority, perhaps 85 per cent, of carers are women (EOC 1980). Recent indications are that a higher proportion of men may be involved in caring than was thought previously (Twigg 1992).

It has been established that female carers are likely to be offered less support and practical assistance than men, presumably because of the predominant view that caring comes naturally to women (Wright 1986). This view makes it harder for women to admit that they are finding the task of caring difficult, particularly if their difficulty relates to their ability to provide intimate 'nursing' care.

When women take on a caring role they may have to take responsibility for many aspects of running a household that have been unfamiliar to them; for example, household repairs and maintenance and filling in income tax returns. Similarly, men taking a caring role may have to take over the running of the house and the attendant domestic tasks. The generation that is in its 70s and 80s may have had a very traditional division of labour in their marriages; some older women have never written a cheque or had to negotiate with builders and repair men. On the other hand, men of this generation will have been in the services and will have some experience of looking after themselves.

Many carers are themselves elderly, they may be in poor health and may have had little experience of negotiating help. They are more likely to be economically disadvantaged and less willing to 'make a fuss'.

It is worthwhile reflecting briefly on how the statutory organisations involved in caring view carers; they are often seen as a major resource, being available to provide help and assistance, filling in the large gaps between the services of the agencies. They will on occasions be seen as 'clients' and will all be 'patients'; this may affect their level of involvement in the design and delivery of services. More helpfully they may be viewed as co-workers, where their interests and views are taken account of and where they are given equal status with professionals. At various stages of the caring relationship any one carer may be viewed in each of these roles. No wonder that carers are often baffled and confused about their relationship with caring agencies (Twigg 1992).

THE IMPORTANCE OF THE RELATIONSHIP

There are almost always some problems associated with caring; this should come as no surprise given the issues that need to be resolved – the change in the balance of power in the relationship, the anxiety of the responsibility, the sense of exploitation and the fear of being manipulated (Froggatt 1990). The success of the caring relationship will depend on the quality of the previous relationship and the capacity and resilience of the carer to meet and cope with a range of demands, both physical, mental and emotional (Ungerson 1987). Particular stresses are associated with different groups of carers; for those older carers who are looking after their spouse the greatest danger is often the likelihood of their continuing to be able to carry on caring being taken for granted by professionals. Many carers in this position see caring as a continuation of the commitment to their marriage vows, but many will have the experience of having their endeavours taken for granted by statutory agencies. A survey has found that spouses are least likely to receive supportive services (Green 1988) even though many older husbands and wives will find the giving of intimate care difficult. Husbands and wives who become carers are likely to suffer from a great loss in social contact, their main companion for many years being the person they now care for. Equally important is the fact that they may feel the greatest degree of guilt when they have to ask for help or the person they care for is admitted to a residential unit.

Where sons and daughters are caring for parents they will have to have negotiated some degree of role reversal. The caring, nurturing parent of their childhood becomes the object of their care and the 'inexperienced' child becomes the responsible carer. It appears that there is a difference in the kind of relationship found between sons and daughters caring for their parents. It often seems that the most successful relationship is a son caring for his mother or a daughter caring for her father. The less successful combination is where the child and the parent are of the same gender. This is in spite of the issues of 'cross sex caring' in relationship to incest taboos (Froggatt 1990).

This role reversal usually takes place long after the child has reached maturity, the success of the relationship may depend on whether the child has left home or not. Sons and daughters who have stayed at home may have slipped into the caring role without making a conscious decision and may have no other option but to carry on. In the 'worst case scenario' adult children can lose their homes when a parent has to go into residential care.

In some families a married son will propose caring for his frail parent knowing that the daily burden of care will fall to his wife. This may work well but needs careful negotiation between the couple. An added difficulty may arise if the wife's parents themselves subsequently need assistance.

As professional staff have become more aware of the needs of carers they have tended to forget about those family members who live at a distance and have concentrated on giving help, assistance and support to the local principal carer. It must be borne in mind that the absent family member may have wanted to be the main carer but was prevented from doing so by the constraints of a job or their own family commitments. This family member may have the strongest relationship with the person requiring care and may be feeling the most distressed about not being available. Staff should try to assure them that they fully involve these family members and that they are clear about who, within the family, has the responsibility for making decisions.

NEIGHBOURS AS CARERS

Some older people living alone will be supported by one or more neighbours. The person's chances of being able to remain at home for as long as possible may depend on the understanding, tolerance and goodwill of these neighbours. Staff working in the community will need to be mindful of the tensions between giving friends and neighbours sufficient information, while protecting the confidentiality of the person needing help. The decision about what information is shared and with whom should not be made by any one individual. It is more appropriate for the decision to be made in the context of a case discussion involving the person's family or advocate and key worker.

WHY DO THEY DO IT?

If one considers the verb 'to care', it has a dual meaning of 'providing physical assistance' and 'being concerned'. These two elements of 'feeling' and 'doing' are always present in any caring relationship, in different proportions. For some people the actions of caring take place within a loving relationship, in others it survives in spite of the absence of positive feelings.

Some carers will have made a positive choice to offer either physical assistance, emotional or financial support or accommodation; others will have had no real option but to provide each aspect of care. People's sense of duty and of what is right may have been influenced by the reality that the family's current and future finances could be seriously affected if an elderly relative has to sell their house and go into care. Some carers will have found themselves 'selected' either by the person needing care or by the wider family. Their selection may often relate more to their availability than their suitability for the task. Others will have drifted into the situation, often accepting responsibility in the short term without appreciating the ramifications of their decision. There is never a simple rationale that accounts for people taking on the responsibility of care. In most cases there will be a mixture of reasons; feelings of duty, love, stubbornness, the desire to prove something to other family members or the ignorance or rejection of alternative support services.

IS CARING FOR SOMEONE WITH DEMENTIA HARDER THAN CARING FOR SOMEONE PHYSICALLY FRAIL?

There are particular aspects of caring for people with dementia that make the caring task more problematic. In the early stages of the disease the carer's role may be mainly supervisory, with only the minimum of physical assistance being required. However, even in these situations the carer will be in a situation where, day by day, little by little, they are forced to accept the deterioration of the person they care for. Obviously many carers are faced with a deteriorating situation but in dementia there is the added difficulty that the personality of the person with the illness is changing and deteriorating. As the disease progresses there is an increased likelihood of the carer having to provide physical and emotional support and the carer is faced with a variety of losses. They may have lost a sense of companionship, they may not have any positive feedback from, and they may not be recognised by, the person they care for. In addition they may have withdrawn from any involvement in their community or wider family circle in order to 'protect' the person they care for.

Carers have described the situation as a 'living death'; they are suffering from a partial bereavement yet still have to care for the 'body'. The individual tasks involved in caring may not be a problem in themselves but the unremitting nature of the need for care, the wide range of extra responsibilities involved and the changes that occur in the relationship as a result of the disease conspire to make caring for someone with dementia a particularly difficult job (Levin, Sinclair and Gorbach 1989). As if this were not enough, the person needing care may have a complete lack of insight into their problem and may not accept the need for care.

WHAT IS THE COST OF CARING?

For many people the decision to take on the role of carer may involve them in giving up their paid employment, moving house and forgoing many of their previous pleasures. The stresses that carers perceive in their role will be related to their individual situations, to their tolerance and to the strength of the relationship (Braithwaite 1990). Research has shown some aspects of care that are particularly associated with stress (Levin, Sinclair and Gorbach 1989; Nolan and Grant 1989). This research highlights the way in which different 'problems' impacted on carers. It found, for example, that one of the more difficult aspects of care to cope with was the prospect of disturbed nights, yet surprisingly few statutory agencies have attempted to provide a service which would assist with this. It is not uncommon for some carers to get up three or four times a night, every night of the week, to assist the person they care for.

Many carers suffer from ill health themselves as a direct consequence of their caring role. They may have hurt their back while lifting, they may be suffering from a stress-related disorder or may be permanently exhausted. In a recent survey half the carers of people with dementia reported that they spent more than 80 hours a week caring (ADS 1993).

The Alzheimers Disease Society report *Deprivation and Dementia* found that 20 per cent of carers aged more than 80 years were spending more than £300 a month on funding care and 41 per cent of carers had drawn on their savings or taken out a loan or sold property in order to meet the cost of caring. Many carers are reluctant to apply for benefits, seeing them as charity (Richardson, Unell and Aston 1989). Application forms are often complex and carers who have been 'careful' and who have accumulated savings may find themselves ineligible for some means-tested benefits.

Resources available to help carers will vary from area to area. To make life more complicated the charging policies and criteria for access will vary and carers will have to negotiate their way around the services provided by the Health Authority, Social Services and Primary Health Care team.

WHAT MAKES THEM STOP

It is clear that many older people with dementia are admitted to care not because of a substantial change in their circumstances but because of a change in the ability of the older person or in the tolerance of their carers (Challis and Davies 1986; Zarit, Todd and Zarit 1986). It is clear that certain difficulties seen in dementia contribute more to carers giving up than others; many carers report the difficulty of managing day after day when one's sleep is constantly disturbed (Chenoweth and Spencer 1986), while others find more difficulty with the inability of the person they care for to recognise them and understand their relationship to them.

The quality, quantity and ease of access of alternative care may affect how carers feel about 'giving up'. Where facilities are perceived to be poor carers will carry on, in spite of difficulties; where facilities are good and easy to access carers may feel more confident about allowing the person they care for to enter care (Hunter, McKeganey and MacPherson 1988).

CONFLICTS OF INTEREST

There is often a difference of opinion between the carer and the person they care for. Often this will be caused by the lack of insight of the older person, who may disagree about the need for assistance, about the risks involved in certain activities and the need for certain supportive services. Staff may find themselves trying to arbitrate and there are circumstances where it may be more appropriate for the older person and the carer to each have a member of staff to represent their interests.

For carers there may be times when they have disagreements with the person they care for about very personal issues. It may be that a wife, caring for her dementing husband, is distressed because he insists on a continuing sexual relationship. Professional care staff must be prepared to help carers deal with these issues. They will need to establish a trusting relationship and allow the carer to 'tell their story' at their own pace. Counselling skills are obviously appropriate and all staff should have some training in 'active listening'.

There will be occasions when there are differences of opinion between staff and carers. These may centre around criticisms by carers of the care provided in an establishment or relate to criticisms that staff may have about the care provided by the carer at home. In either case staff need to be aware of their own feelings and be sensitive to the feelings of the carer while ensuring that the needs of the older person with dementia are given priority. There must be sufficient time for discussion in order that problems can be aired and an attempt made to resolve them. Care staff should ensure that carers are aware of the complaints procedure and managers should ensure that all staff know to whom to report concerns about a person's care at home.

Families may disagree about when it is appropriate for someone to enter full-time care. Even if there is agreement about the timing, there may not be a consensus about the most appropriate establishment. It is not appropriate for a member of staff to 'take over' the decision-making process but staff can ensure that the family has the necessary information and that they can access specialist advice if necessary. There may be situations where the next of kin of the older person is not the main carer; if these two people disagree it may be difficult to ascertain who has the moral right to make the decision. Where staff are involved with people in the early stages of the illness it may be possible to consult them about who should make decisions in the future. Alternatively, the situation may be resolved by the intervention of an advocate.

Within the best functioning team there will be times when staff members have different opinions about the way care is provided. It is important that each staff member has regular supervision from their line manager and that there are times when the staff group can meet together and discuss these issues.

PROFESSIONALS IN PARTNERSHIP WITH CARERS

Helping carers 'let go'

Many carers of people with dementia will have to face allowing the person they care for to enter residential care. This will be a time of great stress and anxiety. No matter how awful the caring situation has become few carers find this situation easy. Staff have a role in supporting people through this period. They may be able to help by assisting the carer to identify that the process they are going through is one of bereavement. As a part of this process staff may need to help the carer deal with their anger and should consider ways of helping the carer plan for 'the rest of their life'. This may involve helping them re-establish a social life, moving to more appropriate housing or obtaining medical or psychiatric help for themselves.

There are a proportion of carers who find it impossible to reach a decision even in the face of the most difficult situations. They may, however, 'listen to the doctor' and it will sometimes be appropriate to ask the consultant or GP to become involved and 'give permission' to the carer to 'let go'.

HOW CAN SERVICES BE ORGANISED TO MAXIMISE THE BENEFIT FOR CARERS?

Day Time Services

The majority of day care and day hospital care operates from 10.30 a.m. to 3.30 p.m.; while there is a belief that a longer day would be too tiring for the user, these 5-hour breaks hardly constitute a 'day off' for the carer. Usually the times of collection and return will be variable so that most carers will find themselves getting home early 'just in case' the transport is early (Murphy 1985).

Staff often encourage carers to use the time to 'enjoy themselves', not appreciating that they may need the time to catch up on chores or sleep, or that they may have lost touch with friends and have nowhere and no one with whom to 'enjoy themselves'. Some day time provision is only available on weekdays and is never open on bank holidays, the very times when carers are the most isolated and the fewest alternative services are available. Some provision finds itself unable to offer care to some people with dementia because they are 'too bad', their physical condition being too frail or their behaviour too unacceptable; yet the carer is expected to carry on coping.

Day time services should ensure that they try to offer a flexible service, open every day of the week. The staff should ensure that transport arrangements are clear and predictable and that wherever possible an escort accompanies the people to and from the centre. This not only helps to allay fears and anxieties but also aids communication between carers and centre staff.

Respite Care

Respite care should be available both in the person's own home and in specially designated units. The most commonly found respite service is one or two beds 'tacked on' to an existing residential or nursing unit. Sometimes the only respite service is found in the occasional use of admission or long-stay beds, when 'deserving cases' are squeezed in, between other admissions.

Many carers are persuaded to use respite care beds only to find that the person they care for comes home substantially worse than when they were admitted. The carer feels guilty and the service is not used again. Often the causes of the change could have been avoided if the staff had had the time to find out more about the person coming into care and the way they were normally looked after.

Carers who are lucky enough to find a respite service that suits the person they care for may find themselves unable to book respite in a pattern that suits them. To be useful respite must be offered before a carer gets to breaking point. The booking process should be as easy as booking into a hotel and it should be possible for the person being admitted to have the same bedroom and be key worked by the same member of staff (Seaborn 1992). Not all carers will want a fortnight's break, not all will want to start the respite period on the same day of the week, the system must be flexible and managers must appreciate that it is not practical to try to obtain 100 per cent occupancy figures in a respite unit.

In many areas respite services will be offered free in a hospital setting and for a charge in a Social Services home. Every effort should be made by staff to ensure that there are clear criteria for each service and that these are clearly understood by fellow professionals.

Staff providing respite services should clarify whether they are trying to provide a rehabilitative or therapeutic environment or whether their aim is simply containment. If rehabilitative-style service is chosen staff must ensure that their views on the merits of rehabilitation are shared by carers. Consider the woman caring at home for her husband, who has often walked out and got lost. She has coped better in the last 6 months as his mobility has declined. Is it helpful for the staff in a respite unit to help him exercise and become more mobile? It may, in fact, decrease the chances of him being able to return home to his wife.

It is not surprising that some carers feel ambivalent about respite services. The chance of some time without the burden of care is welcomed but there is the fear of having to start again and the concern that one may not cope again (Twigg 1992).

What happens to the carer when the person they care for is in respite care? If they take the opportunity to take a complete break, some staff may be tempted to criticise their lack of contact. If, on the other hand, they visit daily for long periods, staff will wonder why the respite admission was needed. There must be an appreciation of the differences in carers and the fact that for some carers there is great relief at not having to provide the physical care but great pleasure at being able to spend time, as a 'visitor', with the person they care for.

Residential and Nursing Care

When someone with dementia who has been looked after at home by a carer is finally admitted to care there are ample opportunities for causing distress. The period surrounding admission will inevitably be one of tension and stress for the carer and the person they look after. Whatever the staff on the unit do and however well they do it, they cannot substitute for the one-to-one attention of the carer at home. Good practice involves trying to minimise the distress as much as possible, by collecting sufficient and appropriate information about the style of care that suits the person and by staff being aware and sensitive to the feelings of the carer.

Take the situation of a daughter, giving up her job and caring for her mother at home for the last 5 years: eventually she has to admit that the care her mother needs is beyond her, the mother is hostile and aggressive and constantly lashing out. An admission is arranged and after settling her mother in the daughter goes home; that evening she rings the unit to ask how her mother is. What does she want to hear? Will it be best to hear that her mother is presenting a management problem to the staff and has had to be heavily sedated? At least it will endorse the daughter's view that the admission was necessary. What if she is told that the mother has settled well as in 'no problem at all'? Will she believe it and if she does, what will it do for her self-esteem? Obviously carers need to know the truth, but staff need to be aware of the impact it will have on the people who are in a stressful situation. All carers can move, during the course of the admission, from a situation where they occupy a central role in the provision of care to one where they are 'standing on the sidelines'. They may have gone, overnight, from being busy with tasks associated with caring for many hours in each 24-hour period to one where they have only themselves to look after. The staff on the unit must be aware of these sudden changes for the carer and must do all they can to make it easy for them to choose their level of involvement. It must be possible for a carer to feel comfortable about being involved on a daily basis in continuing to help care and it must be just as comfortable for the carer who never wants to assist.

It needs to be remembered how painful some family members, friends and carers will find visiting after admission. There is the constant reminder of the fact that the person with dementia is 'bad enough' to need institutional care and probably reminders, in the shape of other residents or patients, of how the course of the illness affects people. Some adult children will be aware of how common illness is and be fearful that they are glimpsing their own future. There are ways of making visiting a more pleasant experience for everyone. Staff can ensure that the person being visited looks their best, that there are opportunities for visitors to take their relative out into the garden or for a short walk. It can be helpful if visitors have access to a kitchen area where they can make their own cup of tea and where, perhaps, small groups of visitors may get to know each other and be of mutual support. Many frequent visitors will be most comfortable if there is something they can do to assist in a general way; perhaps putting away their relative's clean laundry, helping make up a photograph album, or joining in an activity. Where carers live nearby a pattern of frequent but short visits is often best and staff should not feel critical if relatives from afar only stay for a short while. It is easy for staff members to forget that they may feel at ease on the unit, but many visitors will be unaccustomed to seeing groups of people with dementia.

Providing Help at Home

There is often a dilemma for those people who organise services aimed at assisting people in their own home. The services are usually in short supply (Qureshi and Walker 1989) and the manager will have to decide on whom the service should be targeted; on those vulnerable older people who live alone or to help support carers. There is no doubt that home care services are valued by carers (Sinclair et al 1990) not only for the work they do but also for the companionship they offer. They are seen to have a particular role in maintaining a carer's mental health (Levin et al 1989).

Some issues relate specifically to the home care service. Most relate to the dissonance between the needs of users and the style of the 'traditional' service. The home help service was originally developed as a domestic cleaning service and the design of the service still relates, in some areas, to this. The vast bulk of provision is still offered between 9 a.m. and 1 p.m., the average allocation is approximately 2 hours a week and there is still a tendency to offer male carers more assistance than female carers (Twigg 1992). The historical orientation of the service aimed to substitute for the 'female' aspects of care, yet there are many female carers whose greatest needs are help with 'male' tasks: mending fuses, wiring electric plugs and mowing the grass.

To be appropriate for carers the home care service should aim to be flexible, both in the time it offers the service and in the tasks it undertakes. The staff involved in the service should aim to arrive punctually and their managers should ensure that 'substitute' workers are always available if the usual staff member is away sick or on holiday. There must be an acknowledgement that carers often need help with getting the person they care for out of bed in the early morning and assistance later in the evening at bed time. Home carers must be skilled in the provision of personal care and the help they provide must be integrated into the overall 'package of care'. It may be that a carer would be able to make use of a day centre service if the home help could call early enough to assist in the process of getting the older person ready for the transport.

Notoriously, the local authority home help budget has been the first to be cut when money is tight. This leaves the managers of the service to trim back an hour here and there in order to save the requisite amount of money. Senior managers must be aware of the impact this has on carers, in particular the way it affects the credibility of the service.

THE COMMUNITY NURSING SERVICE

Many carers rely heavily on the help and assistance provided by the district nursing service, but it suffers from some of the problems of the home care service. It is usually in short supply and therefore 'rationed' by the managers; staff are often not in a position to ensure that they can arrive for any specific user punctually. The difficulties arise from the demands on the service to provide intensive care to people acutely ill at home and a more support-focused service for people with a chronic illness. District nurses are in an important position; while providing nursing care at home they are in the ideal position to monitor the care situation and are well placed to give carers advice about specific nursing issues, for example in the management of continence and pressure areas and how to lift safely (Twigg 1992).

The short supply of district nursing often means that carers have no other choice but to undertake 'nursing' tasks themselves and there is a continuing debate about the differences and similarities between the home care service and the district nursing service. In some areas this debate has led to endless arguments about medical baths and social baths, often leaving carers with no service at all. In other areas the managers of the respective services have worked together to analyse the needs of the local community and find a way of providing an integrated service.

In most localities the vast majority of the Health Visitor's time is taken up with providing a service to the 'under fives' and it is unusual for them to be involved in the care of older people. There would be great benefit for carers if this group of skilled staff could be available to them, particularly as they could focus on prevention of further deterioration, education and training and unlike district nurses do not require there to be a specific problem before they can be involved.

SITTING SERVICES

Over the last decade there has been an expansion in the availability of 'sitting services'. The most well known, country wide service, is perhaps that provided by the Crossroads Care Attendants scheme, but in many areas there are smaller schemes where care is provided either by paid workers or by volunteers. Sometimes these services will have been specifically set up to provide help for the carers of people with dementia, in other places the scheme will offer help to any carer. Usually the service is free to the user and most commonly offers an hour or two of 'sitting' a week. Carers speak highly of these services and long waiting lists for help often support this view.

There are some carers who are reluctant to use the service and this may relate to the perceived skill of the sitter. Where services rely on volunteers it is perhaps understandable that carers may be concerned that an 'amateur' will not know what to do (May, McKeganey and Flood 1986). It is necessary for the agency to ensure that carers are aware of its commitment to training and that services are organised in such a way that carers have the opportunity to both tell and show the sitter how they provide care. Sitting services also need to be clear whether they exist primarily to support carers or whether they have a wider role in trying to reduce the isolation of some older people, whether the sitter will just 'keep an eye' on someone while the carer is out, or whether they will try to ensure that they provide an interesting and stimulating time to the person with dementia. Services will need to clarify with their staff what tasks they are able to undertake and be prepared to ensure that the staff have the necessary skills and equipment to be able to provide more than a minding service.

SOCIAL WORK AND COUNSELLING

It seems obvious that, given the stresses of caring, a proportion of carers will require counselling support (Gilliard and Wilcock 1993). It might also seem apparent that social workers are well placed both to provide this counselling support and assist in the organisation of practical assistance. However, few qualified social workers work with older people and fewer still with people who have dementia. Until the advent of the NHS and

Community Care Act many social workers felt that working with older people was less interesting and less demanding than child care and an involvement with services for older people could seriously damage their chances of progressing to more senior ranks (Marshall 1983). Since April 1993 many social workers have taken on the role of assessor and care manager. While it is of great help for carers to have a named person in charge of their 'package of care' the move has done little to improve the availability of 'social work'. Social workers in their care management role can now 'buy in' a range of services from the private and independent sector. This kind of work will require additional skills and knowledge and it may be some considerable time before workers have the confidence and expertise to mobilise a range of creative services on behalf of their clients.

Social work managers should ensure that the systems used in the department will allow and facilitate social work staff keeping in touch with carers. All too often the pattern of work demanded by the organisation is one of short-term intervention, whereas it is clear that carers feel unsupported if they are aware that their 'case' is being opened and closed and that at the time of their next crisis they may be allocated a new worker who has little knowledge of them.

COMMUNITY PSYCHIATRIC NURSES

Obviously there are a range of professionals who can supply counselling, support and information. One of the main groups of staff in this position will be community psychiatric nurses, for whom this will comprise one aspect of their clinical role (Adams 1989). In many ways these staff face similar problems to social workers and district nurses, in that they work under pressure and have to balance the needs of people with chronic problems against the needs of people who are acutely ill. People with dementia are more likely to get a high quality service where specialist teams of workers exist who can focus on older people and develop appropriate skills and knowledge.

SUPPORT GROUPS

At the same time that professional care staff discovered carers they also discovered support groups and recognised that they may be an appropriate intervention. Many groups are now provided for and by carers across the country. These groups fulfil a vital role, providing information and support as well as a social outlet for isolated carers. It must be recognised that support groups are not appropriate for everyone (Wilson 1986). At their best these groups can empower carers and ensure that they are involved in the planning of future services.

Setting up a carers' group requires careful planning; groups rarely 'just happen', they need to be fostered and supported and this usually implies professional support (Richardson et al 1989). Any professional contemplating starting a group must be clear about their objectives for the group and must also clarify the extent to which they are prepared to stay involved; the commitment of a professional worker to the group will help to ensure that it stays focused. The style of the group must be matched to the needs of the carers involved. Some will prefer an informal meeting, some a structured programme, others will want to feel able to let off steam while others may be primarily looking for information.

THE NEEDS OF ETHNIC MINORITY CARERS

The number of carers from ethnic minority groups is not known (Squires 1991) but there is evidence that they are substantially disadvantaged (Norman 1985). People who provide services to older people need to be aware of the different beliefs, attitudes and philosophies to old age, illness and caring that are to be found among people from different ethnic backgrounds. It appears that few carers from ethnic minority groups make use of support services (Richardson et al 1989) and this has been used to justify the commonly held belief that there is little need for services for older people from these ethnic groups because 'they all live in extended families and look after their own'. It is far more likely that the services are not used because they are not known about or are not seen as appropriate.

Information for carers should be available in an appropriate form. If one is working in an area with only a small proportion of older people from ethnic backgrounds it is easy to overlook the need for leaflets to be printed in a variety of languages. Staff need to be aware of language difficulties, especially during the course of dementia; people may lose the ability to speak in anything except their mother tongue. In addition to language problems, staff need to ensure that ethic minority users will not be subjected to racist remarks from other users and that the food and bathing arrangements meet the users' requirements.

In some areas it will be more relevant for a statutory agency to contract for support services with a provider who can provide staff from similar backgrounds to potential users.

THE IMPACT OF THE NHS AND COMMUNITY CARE ACT

One of the underpinning philosophies of the NHS and Community Care Act was that carers should be involved in the design of care packages and that their needs should be taken into account. How this is to be achieved will vary from authority to authority, but some Social Services departments, as the lead agency, have designed an assessment format that encourages assessors to ask carers about their needs. The patterns of care emerging in the first few months after April 1993 indicated that, as might have been predicted, fewer people were entering residential and nursing care than in the previous year. If more people are being maintained at home it is inevitable that an additional burden is falling on carers. It is to be hoped that there is a steady increase in the range and quantity of supportive services but it will take some time for alternative services to be developed and for staff to be familiar and comfortable with using them.

Under the new funding arrangements third party 'top-ups' are still permitted, in order to allow someone to access residential care in a setting where the Social Services department would not normally be able to meet the cost. While this gives some carers the flexibility to choose a particular home it may lead to some people feeling obliged to provide substantial amounts of money weekly in order to obtain an acceptable service. Where a person with dementia is assessed as needing residential or nursing care the local authority should provide sufficient funds to enable an appropriate place to be secured.

Social Services departments also have the responsibility for drawing up the Community Care plan for their area. It is increasingly common for carers to be involved both in the drafting of these plans and in the consultation process. It is imperative that these planning groups are able to continue to involve carers and that they hold meetings at suitable times, in accessible places and that they reimburse the carer for the costs of attending the meeting. The people with the responsibility for chairing these planning groups should also ensure that the carer representative feels able to participate fully in the discussion. This may mean being prepared to brief them prior to the meeting, preparing background reading for them and ensuring that other members of the group do not use meaningless jargon.

STAFF AS CARERS

People who manage services must be aware that their staff are 'carers' and although they are rewarded for their efforts and only 'care' in 8-hour shifts, they may be subject to all of the stresses found in carers. In particular there may be occasions when staff are also in the role of carers in their private lives. There is a need for staff to be able to access support and to have the opportunity to talk about how their experiences of caring may impact on their working lives.

HELPING CARERS FACE THE DEATH AND BEREAVEMENT

Staff who work with older people are usually aware of many of the issues surrounding death and dying. When looking after someone with dementia who is dying, the issues may be complicated by a mixture of feelings. There can often be a great sense of relief that the end is in sight and some carers will have done a substantial amount of preparatory grieving. Where the death is expected, and the person has been known to the service for some time, there should have been an opportunity for staff to sense how the carer is feeling and how best to support them. Some will want to be closely involved with the care of their loved one as they near death, others will choose to say their goodbyes and be more distant. Staff must not be judgemental or make assumptions about how carers will react.

Many people with dementia will suffer from chest infections as they become more impaired; many carers will wish to indicate how they feel about the active treatment of such illnesses and when these preferences are expressed they should be recorded carefully.

There is much that staff can do to make the situation easier for carers. They can ensure privacy, can provide practical help and support and can be sensitive to the wishes of the family after the death. It is never appropriate, no matter how urgently the bed is required, to bundle up the dead person's belongings into plastic sacks ready for collection. Carers must be consulted, they must decide who collects the property and when this is done.

Carers may appreciate the attendance at the funeral of staff members and some carers will want to keep in touch with the staff group, if only for a short while. Staff groups may decide to write or telephone bereaved carers, or invite them to functions within the unit and some units will be able to provide bereavement counselling; some carers will welcome these offers, while others will choose to sever all connections.

THE IDEAL SITUATION

Carers around the country seem to have similar views about their general needs. They often put the need for good information at the top of their 'wish list' (WHO 1989). A preference is also expressed for a single access point for services and the right to have a named contact. Carers also rate highly the need for sufficient, high quality respite care and their preference is for the service to be provided in small dedicated units.

Carers are frequently not fussy about who provides a service, or the exact qualifications of the provider. They are always concerned that the service is appropriate and of a high quality. It is imperative that staff in nursing and medical services and in Social Services departments learn to work closer together, sharing training opportunities and developing a close and trusting relationship in every locality. Managers of each service should be involved in the design of each other's services and be able to ensure that the services appear 'seamless'. Wherever possible a 'joint commissioning' approach should be considered.

ACTION FOR CHANGE

1. Design a training programme that will ensure that the staff are 'carer aware'. Involve carers and carers' organisations in the programme.
2. Consider your policies from the carer's point of view, invite carers to comment on them and undertake to include carers in the formulation of all future policy.
3. Look at the ways you give information to carers; are they appropriate (in plain English, in large enough print, available in translations, etc.)? Devise a system where you continually monitor their effectiveness.
4. Ask the carers you know where they go for information. Ensure that wherever they mention has up to date information about the services available in their area.
5. Use a simple questionnaire to collect the views of carers who use the various services you offer, about how easy they are to access and whether the style of the service meets their need. Ask your local university or polytechnic for assistance on the design of the questionnaire. For an example see Jones (1990).
6. Organise opportunities for staff members to spend time at home learning what life is like for carers. Ensure that the visit is for long enough to give them a real flavour of the difficulties that carers face. Build this in to every new staff member's induction programme.

7. Set up a carers' support group or give assistance to existing groups by offering accommodation for meetings, helping with transport or looking after people while carers attend. If in doubt consult the Alzheimer's Disease Society about how to set up a group (Gordon House, 10 Greencoat Place, London SW1P 1PH).

REFERENCES

Adams T (1989) Dementia and family stress. *Nursing Times* **85**(38): 27–29.

Alzheimer's Disease Society (1993) *Deprivation and Dementia.* London: Alzheimer's Disease Society.

Braithwaite V (1990) *Bound to care.* Sydney: Allen and Unwin.

Challis D and Davies B (1986) *Case management in Community Care.* Aldershot: Gower.

Chenoweth B and Spencer B (1986) Dementia: the experience of family caregivers. *The Gerontologist* **26**(3): 267–72.

Equal Opportunities Commission (1980) *The experience of caring for Elderly and Handicapped Dependants: Survey Report.* Manchester: Equal Opportunities Commission.

Froggatt A (1990) *Family Work With Elderly People.* London: Macmillan.

Gilliard J and Wilcock G (1993) Counselling for the carers. *Elderly Care* **5**(1): 24–26.

Green H (1988) *General Household Survey 1985: Informal Carers.* London: HMSO.

Hunter D, McKeganey N and MacPherson I (1988) *Care of the Elderly.* Aberdeen: Aberdeen University Press.

Jones C A (1990) Respite care: A carer's dream come true? *Care of the Elderly* **2**(8).

Kelling K (1993) The cost of caring. *Nursing Standard* **7**(42): 22–23.

Levin E, Sinclair I and Gorbach P (1989) *Families, Services and Confusion in Old Age.* Aldershot: Gower.

Marshall M (1983) *Social Work with Older People.* London: Macmillan.

May D, McKeganey N and Flood M (1986) Extra hands or extra problems? *Nursing Times* **82**(36): 35–38.

Murphy E (1985) Day care: who and what is it for? *New Age* **31**: 7–9.

Nolan M and Grant G (1989) Addressing the needs of informal carers: a neglected area of nursing practice. *Journal of Advanced Nursing.* **14**(11): 959–61.

Norman A (1985) *Triple Jeopardy: Growing Old in a Second Homeland. Policy Studies on Aging No 3.* London: Centre for Policy on Ageing.

Parker R (1990) *Further analysis of the 1985 General Household Survey Data on Informal Care: Report 1. A Typology of Caring.* York: Social Policy Research Unit University of York.

Qureshi H and Walker A (1989) *The Caring Relationship.* London: Macmillan.

Richardson A, Unell J and Aston B (1989) *A New Deal for Carers.* London: King's Fund Centre.

Seaborn A (1992) Making a break. *Nursing Times.* **88**(42): 44–45.

Sinclair I, Parker R, Leat D and Williams J. (1990) *The Kaleidoscope of Care: A Review of Welfare Provision for Elderly People.* London: HMSO.

Squires A (1991) *Multicultural Health Care and Rehabilitation.* London: Edward Arnold.

Twigg J (ed.) (1992) *Carers Research and Practice.* London: HMSO.

Ungerson C (1987) *Policy is Personal: Sex, Gender and Informal Care.* London: Tavistock.

Wilson J (1986) *Self Help Groups – Getting Started, Keeping Going.* London: Longmans.

World Health Organisation (1989) *Health of the Elderly. Technical Report Series 779.* Geneva: WHO.

Wright F (1986) *Left alone to care.* England: Gower.

Zarit S, Todd P and Zarit J (1986) Subjective burden of husbands and wives as caregivers: A longitudinal study. *The Gerontologist* **26**(3): 260–66.

8 The Philosophy of Care
Ethical issues and moral dilemmas

People working in the caring professions are constantly confronted with issues which have no simple answer or, if they do have an answer, it is unpalatable either for the client, the carer or the professional and so leads to lack of discussion. It is important to debate issues relating to the care of people with dementia as openly and positively as dilemmas are debated for any other client group. For some staff who have become entrenched in care-giving on a routine daily basis, it may be difficult to stop and analyse the arguments surrounding treatment methods, approaches to clients, or attitudes to social issues.

This chapter will concentrate on the more philosophical approaches to care delivery. Within many of the areas discussed answers will not be offered; by the nature of the subject this would be inappropriate. By the end of this chapter it is hoped that the reader will be able to consider issues that affect their every activity from a more analytical perspective, and thus from a more objective one.

POINTS TO PONDER

- Stand back and consider how people are cared for in your unit. Would you like to be managed in that way?

- Have you ever been sitting in a car with a seat belt on and find you cannot undo it? What did it feel like?

- Think about your client group; has there ever been an incident of suspected mistreatment by a carer or professional that was ignored?

- Think about your retirement. Have you organised someone to hold an Enduring Power of Attorney? (Public Trust Office 1994) Did you know that you should?

- Think about your own cultural background. What is precious to you?

- Think about your own sexuality. Think what would be said about your lifestyle by a group of people chatting over a cup of coffee!

- Can you recall the last time any member of staff talked about 'ethics'?

- Could all the staff group describe the principle used to ensure that services are distributed fairly?

All members of the staff team, regardless of professional background and status need to become aware that every 'clinical' decision taken will have an ethical context (Reiser et al 1987). In many staff groups, ethics are rarely, if ever, mentioned; if managers of services for older people really wish to deliver consistent high quality care then they must provide an environment where is is safe for staff to challenge a colleague's opinions and beliefs and to be challenged.

These discussions should examine not only attitudes and beliefs, but also ethical issues and moral dilemmas. Many staff have an antipathy to 'ethics', perhaps recalling a brief introduction to the subject during their studies; they may see it as a 'dry' subject that has little relevance to everyday life. However, ethics can offer two important things to care professionals: it can provide a framework to aid decision-making and can make people more aware of their own value base.

WHAT ARE ETHICS?

Ethics are concerned with how we ought to live our lives and everyone will develop, through their life experience, an individual range of beliefs, principles and standards that form their personal ethical code (Seedhouse 1988). Few people are able easily to give an account of the ethical perspective they hold but it will inform all of their actions (Brody 1983).

The work that people are involved in when looking after older people will often bring them face to face with difficult moral dilemmas, although not all staff will recognise them as such. It would be naive to suggest that ethical dilemmas usually have straightforward and simple solutions, but discussions can often lead to a better understanding or acceptance of a situation.

The public at large want to feel confident that people in the caring professions are looking after the people in their charge to the best of their ability, and within the constraints of the law are offering older people with dementia autonomy and opportunity of choice. Hillan (1993) argues that this may not be the situation in all care environments and that the demented person is not given the same civil rights as other members of the community to excercise free will. Whether the care professional acts paternally towards the client or ensures complete freedom of choice, even if the person is unaware of their actions, is an ethical dilemma, but the choice is not that simple.

It would be equally naïve to suggest that professional care staff will always identify ethical issues in their daily practice and they may find it difficult to think of situations that illustrate ethical or moral problems. As a starting point it is often helpful, instead, to ask staff members to reflect on situations at work that make them angry, or sad, or feel powerless; these situations will frequently have an 'ethical' dimension to them.

THE RELATIONSHIP OF PRINCIPLES, GUIDELINES AND LAWS TO ETHICS

The majority of staff who are offering care to older people with dementia will have access to a range of 'principles', 'codes of practice', 'good practice guidelines' or 'operational instructions'; while all these statements have value they do not provide 'off the shelf' solutions for every moral dilemma. Consider the 'five ethical issues' as outlined by the United Kingdom Central Council (UKCC 1992). They are described as being relevant to all caring situations and are: beneficence, non-maleficence, fidelity, autonomy and equity. They are not necessarily words that turn up in everyday conversation, but they do apply to difficulties that arise daily in caring situations, giving direction to how staff can think about and attempt to resolve problems. It may be helpful to think further about each of these five qualities and what they may mean for daily practice.

Beneficence is 'the intention to do good' and is perhaps the easiest to identify with. For many care staff the intention to do good will be achieved through 'looking after people', yet there will be many occasions where 'good care' involves *not* 'doing things' for people but standing back and letting them do tasks for themselves, even where this takes longer, achieves a lower standard and involves some degree of risk.

Non-maleficence is 'the intention not to knowingly cause harm'. Few care professionals will consider that they are ever involved in harmful care practices, yet there are occasions when people are given medication not so much for its therapeutic effect but for the peace of the staff. In other situations staff seriously undermine older people's confidence and feelings of self-worth by a thoughtless or offhand remark about their ability, dexterity or mobility.

Fidelity can be described as an allegiance and faithfulness to the older person's best interests. It involves acting as advocate for the older person and always representing their interests even when this may involve staff in additional work or conflict with people.

Autonomy involves asserting the right of the older person to maximum liberty and freedom. It involves staff in being able to analyse carefully and balance risks against rights. It also requires staff to allow older people with dementia to take as much responsibility as possible and to involve the older person in decision-making wherever possible.

Equity requires staff to offer the same quantity and quality of care to all people regardless of their origins, gender, age, religion or sexual orientation. It means that older people who are less grateful, more aggressive, less 'lovable' or dirtier should receive the same care as those who are grateful, gentle and socially acceptable. It means that even the most demented person should be able to access any medical or social care that they require and that no one should be excluded from treatment of a physical illness because of the degree of their mental deterioration.

These five points are very similar to Thiroux's Principles, quoted in Tschudin (1986), in that they form a useful starting place for discussing ethical issues and a checklist of standards that actions can be measured against, but they do not suggest either a process or formula that can assist a staff group to resolve an ethical problem.

Before presenting a way of assisting staff to participate in ethical debates it may be helpful to clarify the difference between morality and legality (Seedhouse 1988). An action can be immoral but not illegal; an example of this may be the disclosing of confidential information. It is also possible to argue that some activities can be moral but illegal. The best example of this may be the turning of a 'blind eye' while a trusted relative 'forges' a signature on a pension book because the older person refuses to sign it themselves and no other alternative processes have been put into place.

GETTING STARTED: STRATEGIES FOR RESOLVING DILEMMAS

A simple starting point for a group of staff could be to adopt the maxim 'do as you would be done by'. This adage has the advantage of being both well known and easy to understand. It encourages staff to 'put themselves in the shoes' of the person with dementia and to begin to base their decisions on the values and principles that they would want applied to themselves. This simple exercise can have profound effects; over the years many unsatisfactory care practices have been justified on the basis that people with dementia are somehow different and of less value than other people. It is not uncommon for staff to be involved in trying to reach a decision whether an older person with confusion should remain at home or be persuaded to enter residential care. Considering the advantages and disadvantages of each action as if you were the older person can bring a different perspective to the discussion.

This maxim can be of less help where there is more than one person involved in a situation, perhaps the older person with dementia and their carer. Each person's needs and best interests may be in conflict and the staff member may find themselves striving to identify with and champion the causes of both parties.

In situations such as this a different strategy is needed, one that can deal with two conflicting conditions (Brody 1983). Each condition or situation may be governed by 'rules' that seem reasonable but that are mutually exclusive. A familiar example would be the situation where the following 'rules' or principles are in conflict: 'all carers should have a regular break from caring' and 'everybody admitted to a respite service must have agreed to the admission'. In situations involving conflicting needs or wishes one of the simplest ways to begin to evaluate the ethical dimension is to make a judgement about the consequences of adhering to each 'rule' in turn, so rather than trying to rate which 'need' takes priority, the focus is switched to determining the 'best outcome' (Rumbold 1989).

This, hopefully, should lead some staff to think about how, and by whom, 'the best outcome' is defined.

An even more comprehensive way of examining ethics is as a matrix or grid (Seedhouse 1988). Each element of the grid is designed to remind staff of key issues that need to be considered in any debate on ethics. It could be a useful team-building exercise for staff teams to construct their own 'ethical grid' and agree to use it as a template or checklist against which difficult decisions are made.

The rest of this chapter seeks to present some common situations and highlight the underlying ethical issues that ought to be discussed before decisions and actions can be formulated.

BUT SHE'LL WANDER OUT AND GET KNOCKED OVER!

Mrs Jones is moderately confused; she lives in a large residential home in the centre of a busy urban area. The majority of residents in the home are physically frail. Mrs Jones often believes that she still has school-age children and that she needs to go and collect them from school. At these times she is often reported by staff to be 'trying to leave the building'. Beyond the small front garden is a busy main road. The front door of the home is kept unlocked but staff are concerned that Mrs Jones will 'escape' and try to cross the road and cause an accident; they have started lobbying the home owner 'to do something about the situation'. Their preferred options are either to lock the door or sedate Mrs Jones. The proprietor of the home has resisted adopting either of the staff's suggestions so far and is particularly anxious not to lock the front door because of the effect it will have on other residents and their visitors. The key questions that need to be discussed are as follows.

What are Mrs Jones's needs?

It could be argued that Mrs Jones does not ask to be kept safe. Her greatest need may be for continued reassurance, manifested by her concern about her 'children'. The proprietor and their staff will need to consider if they are able to offer this reassurance or whether the home is inappropriate for Mrs Jones. It may be that the layout of the home and the staffing levels are not appropriate for people with confusion, in which case is it ethical to impose restrictions on Mrs Jones because of the 'shortcomings' of the home? If the door is locked or Mrs Jones sedated are the staff demonstrating beneficence?

What is the prime function of the care staff?

Is the prime function to encourage Mrs Jones's autonomy or to protect her? In this situation these two functions seem to be diametrically opposed. One answer could be to seek a middle way, to neither support absolute autonomy nor seek maximum safety.

People have a right to freedom of movement; in extreme situations, where this freedom is restricted or removed without legal justification, there could be a charge of unlawful imprisonment; yet staff are expected to have a 'duty of care' and common law allows staff to act 'in the best interests' of a person who lacks the mental capacity to make their own decisions (Dimond 1993). This may be an occasion when the maxim 'do as you would be done by' is useful.

What is the risk to Mrs Jones?

Are the staff displaying fidelity when they describe the risks to Mrs Jones? It would be necessary to know if Mrs Jones has ever walked out of the home and if she has, has anyone watched her to see how far she ventures? There needs to be an up-to-date assessment of her 'road sense' and a discussion of the situation with Mrs Jones and with her family. This discussion needs to include an assessment of the risks if medication is used to try to change Mrs Jones's behaviour or if a move to another home is recommended (Norman 1980).

How can potential harm be minimised?

The staff have a responsibility both to Mrs Jones and to all of the other residents. This will involve tensions and conflicts which need to be reconciled. Locking the door will affect all the residents, while it could be argued that sedating Mrs Jones will only affect her. Wherever a resolution to a problem can be said to be 'for the greater good', it usually involves a substantial reduction of at least one person's rights.

There will be a range of ways in which a higher degree of safety can be assured for Mrs Jones which should be explored before accepting a 'greater good' type of solution. Some solutions will be more feasible than others and care professionals should be clear about who will 'benefit' most from the solution.

It may be helpful to consider the notion of 'net good'; this approach looks at the good outcomes of any decision and subtracts the negative outcomes, the remainder being the 'net good'. The main drawback to this method of decision analysis is that staff need to ascribe a subjective value to each predicted outcome, so not only may the predictions not happen, but different staff may see outcomes in a different way. A rather exaggerated example may be that one negative outcome of Mrs Jones wandering may be that she is killed in a road accident. Some staff may see this as a great misfortune, others as a timely release from a terminal illness.

What is the best outcome for Mrs Jones?

Is it preferable for Mrs Jones to be moved to a home better able to keep her safe, or is it better for her to stay in familiar surroundings? Is it better for Mrs Jones to live the rest of her life frustrated because she is kept locked in or is it better for her to feel some sense of freedom but be knocked over by a car in a few months' time?

Quality of life should take preference over quantity of life and staff need to understand that questions involving the words 'better' or 'preferable' need close analysis – the questions 'better for whom?' and 'preferable from whose perspective?' need to be asked. Many care staff are already familiar with the concept of 'quality of life'; while it is a helpful concept there needs to be an understanding that no one can fully appreciate what constitutes quality in someone else's life (Rumbold 1989).

SHE CAN GO IF SHE WANTS TO, I'LL BE ALL RIGHT ON MY OWN

Mr and Mrs Smith have been married for 55 years. Mr Smith has dementia and is cared for by Mrs Smith with the minimum of outside help. Mrs Smith has found the last few months extremely hard and her physical health is suffering. Her daughter has arranged for Mrs Smith to fly out to the USA to see her youngest son. The plan depends on Mr Smith agreeing to go into a residential unit for 2 weeks' respite care. Mr Smith is refusing to go and thinks he can manage on his own at home. Mrs Smith is desperate to have the break but will not leave her husband at home alone. Mr Smith is also refusing to have someone 'live in' or call daily.

Is it appropriate that professional care staff are involved in this decision between husband and wife?

Are there some situations that can only be resolved within the family or is it appropriate for professionals to try to 'arbitrate'?

When people disagree it is common for each of them to state their case in terms that are completely 'black and white'. The role of the professional may be to help them examine the 'shades of grey' in between. Caring for older people is not like a pure science based on provable facts and certainties; the work involves human feelings and has to be based on probabilities. In situations of conflict it is helpful for the professional to assist each of the parties to engage together in discussions which lead to a decision that both parties can live with (Reiser et al 1987).

The person facilitating such a discussion needs to be aware that each of the parties has an equal right to express their wishes but that if one of them is intellectually failing they may be disadvantaged when presenting their argument. If the facilitator takes on the role of advocate, they must be mindful that their remit is to help the person with dementia make their *own* case (Yeo 1991).

Whose needs should predominate?

It would appear that Mr and Mrs Smith have expressed conditions that are mutually exclusive. If Mr Smith's autonomy is to be preserved then his wishes must not be assumed to be less important than those of his wife. It is useful to consider if the needs that they describe are real 'needs' or whether they are better thought of as 'wants'.

It could be argued that Mr Smith *needs* assistance and that Mrs Smith *needs* a break, Mrs Smith *wants* to go to America and Mr Smith *wants* to stay at home. If the situation is reframed like this, it is possible to see that both sets of needs could be satisfied by providing intensive or live-in assistance for Mr Smith and let Mrs Smith rest at home. Once the basic needs have been satisfied one can start to look at ways of meeting people's 'wants'; in this situation, perhaps the son could visit his parents.

HE'D GIVE THE WINDOW CLEANER A CHEQUE FOR £100 IF ASKED

Mr Allen is a confused, elderly man living alone in a large detached house full of valuable antiques. He is a retired bank manager who has always been obsessively organised. His son has been anxious for some time about his father's ability to look after his own finances. The concern first surfaced when Mr Allen's son visited his father and discovered that his father had put a £50 note into a charity envelope put through the door.

The key worker in the situation has begun to discuss Mr Allen's finances with him. He refuses to see that he is at any risk and constantly emphasises his experience and skill in looking after other people's money throughout his professional career. He is adamant that he will not let anyone else assist him in looking after his finances.

What would individual staff want for themselves in this situation?

If people put themselves in Mr Allen's position they may opt for allowing him to retain control of his finances. Having reached this decision it would be helpful for staff to discuss how much money they would want to be allowed to 'go astray' before the position was reconsidered. Some staff may find the situation easier to resolve if Mr Allen lived on income support, but how can these staff claim to be treating people with equity if the decision depends on the amount of money involved? In addition, any staff who would feel comfortable allowing Mr Allen to take the risk of losing money should reflect on whether they would change their view if they were told that Mr Allen used to often express his exasperation at muddled old ladies who refused to let the bank look after their financial matters. Putting yourself in someone's place is helpful but should not take priority over any information about the person's own view of the world.

How do you assess the risk in this situation?

It may well be possible to argue that Mr Allen's sense of autonomy is best preserved if the risk to property and money is accepted. Imagine for a moment that Mr Allen's choice is to stay at home supported by a live-in companion. Consider the consequences for Mr Allen were he to suffer a series of misadventures with his finances that leaves him without sufficient income to continue to pay for this support. The acceptance of risk may have seemed to be justified because it supported his autonomy, but it could lead to his having a very much more restricted choice in his support systems.

In reality there is a range of actions that could be taken to effect some degree of protection for Mr Allen and his finances. Before a decision can be taken about which is the most appropriate it is necessary for the staff involved to feel confident that they are aware of all of the potential alternatives. No decision can be made without a careful assessment of the problem *and* the gathering of relevant data that can inform the decision-making process. There are several models, including those of Jameton and Crisham, that help lead staff through the process from identification of the problem to planning, implementation and evaluation (Tschudin 1986; Benjamin and Curtis 1992).

A study of ethics can assist staff in their daily routine; it is particularly relevant in situations where services and resources have to be rationed and people's needs prioritised. Professional care staff need to feel that they have dealt with conflicting demands for service fairly. In order to do this the decisions must be based on some principles that stand ethical scrutiny.

Recent years have seen some growth in public and professional awareness that older people may be abused and that there are also problems associated with the restraint of people with dementia. These two issues in particular are worthy of further discussion.

THE ABUSE OR MISTREATMENT OF OLDER PEOPLE – PUBLIC AWARENESS

Abuse of children has been recognised for over 10 years as a phenomenon which occurs throughout society. This horrifying fact was acknowledged by professionals and politicians only after tragedies such as the death of Maria Coldwell were made public. Thereafter strategies, guidelines, education and legislation were all implemented to raise awareness and give professionals a framework to deal with this crime.

Elder abuse, however, despite first being highlighted as a problem in 1975 with the term 'granny bashing', has not captured society's imagination. Energy on abuse has been channelled by the statutory bodies into child abuse, and even the government are slow in accepting the need for active response. In 1991 the Health Minister Virginia Bottomley said 'I don't frankly think that abuse against the elderly is a major problem' (Community Care 1993). The politicians had shifted their opinion slightly by 1993 when Junior Minister John Bowis supported the practice guidelines in *No Longer Afraid* (Tomlinson 1993). This document highlighted the important differences between child and elder abuse, including the relevance of financial motives, a family perception of a negative future and a negative low status stereotype of older people.

AN OVERVIEW OF ABUSE

There is still a significant group of people who are unaware, or who remain blind to the incidence of abuse in both the population as a whole and among professionals. It is important, therefore, to lay the cornerstone about which discussion can be held.

The broad definition of abuse is as follows.

> The physical, emotional, or psychological abuse of an older person by a formal or informal carer. The abuse is repeated and is the violation of a person's human and civil rights by a person or persons who have power over the life of the dependant. (Eastman 1984).

The recognised eight standard categories of abuse are: assault, deprivation of nutrition, administration of inappropriate or deprivation of prescribed drugs, emotional and verbal abuse, sexual abuse, deprivation of help in performing activities of daily living, involuntary isolation and financial abuse (Bennett 1990). The incidence of abuse remains unquantified in the United Kingdom. In the United States work on identifying the prevalence of abuse has been ongoing for the past 10 years and a steady percentage of 3–5 per cent of older people are being identified as being abused (Pillener 1993). Specific state departments have been initiated to research and develop policies and training packages for both carers and professionals. There has also been developmental work in the United States for support systems, offering projects as diverse as a 24-hour help line, a national data collection system and a counselling programme. Most of these are for the abused however, not for the abuser. (Wolf 1993).

In the United Kingdom the information is far less evident. In 1984 Eastman estimated on subjective knowledge and intuition that there may be as many as 5 per cent of the population being abused (Eastman 1984). The most recent survey conducted identified that 10 per cent of carers admitted abuse and 5 per cent of older people reported being abused (Ogg and Bennett 1992). However, these statistics do not identify the specific nature of the disease the older person suffers from. Evidence of abuse is available, but it is often overlooked due to fear, ignorance or lack of priority (Sutton 1992). For black and ethnic minority older people there is very little evidence of abuse. There is nothing to explain the reason for this; it may be due to their cultural or family lifestyles or to the lack of investigation into their needs.

ABUSE OF PEOPLE WITH DEMENTIA IN THE COMMUNITY

As elder abuse slowly becomes accepted as a phenomenon that must be addressed there is, with equal speed, the hunt for the perpetrator or person to blame. Abuse in the community automatically turns attention to the carer and carer stress is quoted as the reason why the carer snaps and slaps their cared-for across the face. The problem in the community is not that simple. People suffering from dementia may exhibit the same behaviour in their own homes as they do in a residential setting. They may wander, shout, express paranoid ideas or urinate in inappropriate places. In a residential setting this behaviour is hard to bear but the care professional can go home after 8 hours and have their own respite. A carer who lives in the home cannot. Constant sleepless nights or household chores can and do increase carer stress. There are also other differences to be considered. If the carer is a spouse or a child they would have known the demented person when they were well and so have family life dynamics to influence their approach to the dependent person. If they have had a long loving relationship this may assist the carer in continuing in their caring role. If, however, they have had a tortuous relationship, perhaps with a history of abuse themselves, they may not even like the dependent person, let alone feel able to carry out intimate care for them (King 1993).

Within the group of family carers abuse can occur because an exhausted carer becomes frustrated and tired and then violent, or at the other end of the continuum there are carers who exploit the vulnerable older person. It is important to identify that there may be carers who abuse the demented person because they have not been informed of a more appropriate method of care and so give inadequate care. Most carers receive little or no training on how to offer physical and psychological care to a person with dementia, and tasks that care professionals perform automatically may seem complicated and unsolvable (Sadler 1989). The psychological management of someone with perseverative conversation requires skill and patience; carers are not given these skills automatically and yet people are expected intuitively to know how to cope. If serious consideration is to be given to the high incidence of abuse of people who have dementia, it should be supported with evidence to show the complexity of the disease and its effect on the whole family.

It must never be overlooked that the carer themselves could become the victim of abuse by the person with dementia. This, as with any other abusing situation, can present in many ways, from the loss of personal liberty due to caring to psychological, physical or sexual abuse, particularly where the person is experiencing some change in their character or exhibiting disinhibitive behaviour. Financial abuse also causes problems for some carers where their partners perhaps always handled the finances and have become suspicious or unable to manage their affairs.

ABUSE OF PEOPLE WITH DEMENTIA IN RESIDENTIAL SETTINGS

To suggest that abuse occurs in residential settings will cause different care professionals to think of different things. Stereotypical views are evident in the media and among the general public about nursing homes, rest homes and social service homes. The controversy of paying for care versus free care at the point of delivery means that the independent sector and social services bear the brunt of criticism.

Institutional abuse can occur in any institution and, sadly, does. Hospitals can be centres of practice that deny people with dementia their basic human rights and opportunities of personal well-being within the constraints of their disease process.

Abuse within residential care settings can, of course, be perpetrated by individual care professionals who perhaps steal or execute physical abuse, and this should be dealt with within the criminal legislation. There is even less evidence to support the incidence of institutional abuse, so anecdotal information or stories of poor practice can only indicate that the problem of habitual abuse is so entrenched in the work practice and culture of the unit that it is often presumed normal acceptable practice and to suggest abuse would cause uproar and disbelief.

Because of the nature of the disease process, people who have dementia often go into institutional care when their cognitive functioning is so poor that they have difficulty in expressing their wishes and individuality. The area of dementia care is demanding and unglamorous and so often is understaffed and underpinned with low morale. This is compounded by staff who may lack relevant up to date knowledge, and so patterns of care develop that ultimately suit the care professional or the institution rather than the client. Examples of how an institution may abuse people are:

a. getting people up at 5.30 a.m.;
b. no personal belongings;
c. lack of choice in meals and poor meal time planning;
d. toileting and washing in public;
e. stock clothing that is rarely changed; and
f. excessive use of cot sides and tip-back chairs (Tomlinson 1993).

Investigation of a random sample of continuing care hospitals visited in 1987 demonstrated that the abuse of older people's human rights was evident in most of the 12 hospitals that were analysed. The study identified that passive abuse was commonplace, and staff had become entrenched in routines and rituals that were for the benefit of the hospital (Tomlinson 1993). Some abuse occurs because of misguided judgements about risks and the protection of vulnerable people. Other incidents of abuse are due to the unacceptable subculture of the institution.

THE ROLE OF THE CARE PROFESSIONAL IN ABUSE

If care professionals are to become active and effective in the protection of older people with dementia the first and most important step forward is to receive adequate training, either individually or in reflective group work, not only in the skills necessary to identify abuse but also in skills to enable management of the situation (Biggs 1993). This training should reflect an understanding of what abuse is and how to recognise it. There should also be guidelines and policies written to help both staff and manager deal effectively with suspected and actual elder abuse. Effective strategies to deal with abuse are, however, only one part of the package that care professionals should develop within institutional and residential settings. Staff must examine every aspect of their care and practice and examine objectively whether this practice is acceptable or is an abuse of the person's dignity, civil liberty or personal status. It is also important that care professionals look at the causation of abuse within domestic settings and not only identify strategies to deal with abuse, but identify methods of prevention by offering appropriate support, education and respite for carers of people with dementia.

As already discussed elder abuse occurs due to a variety of reasons. Accepting that not every carer has the personal capacity to offer 24-hour care, or that they are only interested in personal vengeance or personal gain, needs to be openly discussed within teams, to help acknowledge self-awareness and growth of a professional's ability to deal impartially with any suspected perpetrator. The care professional should also discuss and be able to debate the rights of the demented person to remain in or leave a situation of abuse and when the demented person should be able to choose the type of intervention. People who have dementia are adults with a very special need. To assess and be able to offer a substantiated rationale for actions that care professionals take to intervene in incidents of abuse should be undertaken only by staff with very specific skills.

PROFESSIONAL ACCOUNTABILITY IN TAKING RISKS

Life for any member of society is full of risks. Rules and regulations are made at all levels to guard the population against unnecessary risk from areas that might be outside their control. Policy makers within governments set standards of acceptable risk. The Department of Trade and Industry has responsibility for most consumer products; for example, all major incidents in the public domain are investigated and the avoidable or unavoidable risk is assessed. When seat belts were introduced in the United Kingdom in 1967, there were debates both for their use, as they saved lives, but also against this statutory law as it impinged on people's personal choice and acceptance of personal responsibility.

Care professionals tend to concentrate on the inabilities of the person rather than their abilities, particularly if an older person is felt to be unable to make rational decisions due to dementia. In one study, social workers were found to express concern about dangers and potential problems even though the older people had not been assessed about their level of risk and they were cognitively intact (Wynne Harley 1991). Throughout life a person is continuously undertaking risk assessment. As babies and throughout the early years of life that assessment is carried out by parents. During adolescence and adulthood individuals set their own limits of risk in daily living. Older people who are ablebodied identify two aspects of risk taking: practical, e.g. taking chances, and recreational, e.g. activities which stimulate or offer excitement. Older people trade the benefits of the risk being positive against the possible negative results of their gamble (Wynne Harley 1991). People with dementia have often lost the ability to make judgements about risk and so care professionals or carers have to step in and make value-judgements on their behalf. The skill, however, is to be able to judge when a risk is acceptable and when it is inappropriate. Life is full of risks. Dangers are more often in the eye of the observer rather than the mind of the participant (Wynne Harley 1991). Few would argue about the right of mentally intact older people to determine their own level of acceptable risk taking; the situation is markedly more complex when caring for people with dementia and particularly fraught when considering the care of someone living at home. It may seem eminently sensible to replace dangerous open fires with safe heaters, until one realises that the confused homeowner cannot remember how to light them and dies from hypothermia. It is unfortunate but true that the degree of risk someone can live with may be determined primarily by where they live. If there is a chance that someone may fall asleep with a lighted cigarette the situation is less likely to cause anxiety to the community if they live in a detached bungalow. If they live in a multi-occupied house their immediate neighbours will rightly feel that they have a right to make their concerns felt.

Measuring risk within a residential setting is also complex. A Coroner's report in a newspaper illustrated this. In 1992 an elderly lady was admitted to a general hospital for investigation. She also had dementia. The nurses assessed that she was at risk of falling out of bed and so put up cot sides. They did not have enough staff to observe her and in her confused state she climbed over the cot sides, fell and hit her head on the floor. She died from her injury. The debate, of course, should be about whether the risk was assessed properly and whether the intervention was the most appropriate. Should other action have been taken? Would a mattress on the floor have been more appropriate, as there was knowledge of her agitation? What were the contra-indications for this in her physical condition? The Coroner's verdict was accidental death as the nurses had taken every appropriate action to prevent a tragedy, but sadly it had occurred. In a caring environment for people with dementia the safety of the environment must therefore incorporate the philosophy of preventing harm from unnecessary life risk. Any injury or death occurring to a person with dementia is a tragedy, but the circumstances of that incident must be analysed. Is it acceptable to have stairs in a unit where someone might trip down? Is it acceptable to have a deep unguarded pond in the garden of a unit that cares for dementia sufferers? Is it acceptable to have an open door policy, as someone might wander out and be knocked down by a car? The answer to all of these illustrations could be 'no', it could equally be 'yes', but more importantly it should be 'maybe'. The debate about the assessment of risk and any associated decisions about implementing major changes in a person's lifestyle should not be taken by any single individual. A multidisciplinary approach should be adopted, the family and friends consulted and the reason for the decision documented and reviewed regularly.

'WANDERING', RESTRAINT AND MOBILITY

The question of restraint highlights the potential conflict between upholding basic human rights and maintaining safety (Darby 1990). It has been found that restraints often exacerbate the problem they sought to solve. The only acceptable response is one that looks for individual resolutions. Every unit should have a policy on restraint and staff should be trained in methods of safe restraint (RCN 1992). All instances where restraints have been used should be documented and if doors are locked as a last resort the fact should be recorded by a senior member of staff and reviewed hourly. Where a person with dementia is felt to be regularly wandersome there should be an assessment that attempts to define the reason for the wandering. As soon as care professionals use the term 'wander' it is suggestive that the demented person does not know what they want to do, and so may suggest that the staff are labelling a person's behaviour unnecessarily. Is the person searching for an object or person, is the wandering aimless or focused on trying to find the exit? The assessment should also define the times of day that the problem is worse and examine what staff were doing at the time and how many staff were available.

An analysis of this assessment will inform a way of resolving the problem. The solution for someone who is wandering in an attempt to find their room will be different to the solution for someone who is constantly looking for the way home, or the person who is used to a substantial amount of exercise.

Incidents of wandering often coincide with unstructured time and the amount of wandering can be reduced by introducing more activity into the unit. Staff need to be mindful both of the pejorative connotations of the term 'wandering' and of the fact that people with dementia have a need and a right to be able to move freely and to be alone.

Recent technological developments have given staff the option of electronic tagging. The advocates of tagging will say that it gives residents a greater freedom, the critics of tagging will say that the method is undignified and an excuse for inadequate staffing. The legal situation is unclear. Tagging without consent could be seen as illegal imprisonment. Tagging is designed to be used on confused people who are unlikely to be able to give informed consent. The fact that a person's relative may agree to the tagging does not count in law, there being no clear status for 'consent by proxy' (Counsel and Care 1993). The most advanced tagging systems can monitor people over distances of a quarter of a mile, yet it must be an unusual unit that will let people walk for this distance before dispatching staff to retrieve them. No one disputes the care professional's duty of care; perhaps the most suitable means of ensuring that staff are aware that someone has left or entered the unit is to have all external doors alarmed and linked to the nurse call system.

Restraint of people who have dementia can, however, be far more subtle than refusing exit from a building. The use of tipped back 'geriatric' chairs is becoming less common, but they are still available in some areas. Their use must be discussed openly and they must be used only as a last resort. The benefits to the older person must be clearly thought out, as total confinement in this way is false imprisonment (Dimond 1993). The care professional does have a duty to the older person to safeguard their rights; the benefits to the client must outweigh any organisational benefit, perhaps because of staff shortages. The belief that restraints are used because of staff shortages is, in fact, becoming more of a myth. Within the nursing profession studies are showing evidence to suggest that the main reason for restraining patients would appear to be for the safety and prevention of harm (Ramprogus and Gibson 1991), and that the main cause for concern was that the older person was at risk from injury. Some experts feel that the older person's presentation becomes accepted as the diagnosis; that confusion, for example, is accepted as the norm and final state and not simply a symptom (Norman 1987).

Routines and rituals that affect the person's quality of life and their autonomy are restraints of the most subtle kind. These, as already argued in this book, may develop as a result of the staff and institution's, or community organisation's, needs and so remain unnoticed and unregistered as a method of restraint (Norman 1987). Balancing risk and restraint is a complex ethical dilemma. If a person continually tries to leave a building for reasons that they cannot explain and the staff feel that such a person is in danger of walking into the road, the care professional has a duty of care to the person, and if the professional does not take reasonable precautions to protect the person they could face an action for breach of the duty of care. If, on the other hand, the staff were aware of the dangers and so removed the client's clothing and shoes and locked them in their bedroom, the basic human right of freedom would be violated and a charge of false imprisonment could be brought against them (Dimond 1993). Care professionals must, therefore, be quite clear within their team why restraint has to be used for a particular client, and blanket policies, for example a locked door policy, should be avoided. Good practice must ensure that every person's human rights are upheld. It must also ensure that care professionals protect a demented person from unnecessary risk. A positive way to balance these two issues would be to develop a control and restraint policy. Every type of restraint should be considered under this policy as well as offering legal advice and positive professional practices as an alternative to some putative measures. The least restrictive alternative should be used, and an environment of open discussion and debate be promoted to help staff examine the full ethical and moral dilemma of an action or activity that might have become the norm.

ACTION FOR CHANGE

1. Encourage staff to share an incident where they have been unhappy about the care of the older person and may have suspected abuse. Analyse the care the team would have given, in the light of additional knowledge of abuse, and then compare this with the evidence of the care actually given.

2. Look carefully at the use of restraint in the residential unit. Make a list from the most obvious, i.e. locked doors, to the more subtle, perhaps not allowing access to a telephone, or using medication. Review their use. Is there a balance between risk management and self-determination?

3. Consider the care plan of the clients and identify if specific risk factors are noted on each plan. Is each person's risk analysis done individually or are they batched into the whole unit?

4. Ascertain if the organisation within which your unit works has an abuse policy. Ensure that all staff are aware of it and are able to view caring situations in an informed, balanced way.

5. Introduce the idea of ethics into individual supervision sessions by asking staff to reflect on how they know what is 'right' for the people they care for.

6. Ask each member of staff to imagine that a much-loved member of their family has dementia. Would they allow them to be cared for by the team? Ask them to consider the main reason behind their decision and share the information with the whole staff team.

7. Encourage the open and creative discussion of 'problems' and 'dilemmas'. Put aside time regularly for the discussion. Get staff members to role-play situations (such as that of Mr and Mrs Smith); ask people to play 'devil's advocate' and try to convince their colleagues of an unpopular solution (such as the sedation of Mrs Jones).

REFERENCES

Benjamin M and Curtis J (1992) *Ethics in Nursing*, 3rd edn. Oxford: Oxford University Press.

Bennett G (1990) Action on elder abuse in the '90s, new definition will help. *Geriatric Medicine*, April, 53–54.

Biggs S (1993) Getting in training. *Community Care*, 15 July, 15.

Brody B (1983) *Ethics and its Applications*. New York: Harcourt Brace Jovanovich.

Community Care (1993) A National Scandal. *Community Care*, 6 May, 17–18.

Counsel and Care (1993) *People and not Parcels: A Discussion Document*. London: Counsel and Care.

Darby S (1990) Containing the wanderer. *Nursing Times* 86(15): 42–43.

Dimond B (1993) A case of false imprisonment. *Elderly Care* 5(1): 18–19.

Eastman M (1984) *Old Age Abuse*. London: Age Concern.

Hillan E (1993) Nursing dementing elderly people: Ethical issues. *Journal of Advanced Nursing* 18: 1889–94

King J (1993) Walking a tightrope. *Community Care*, 24 June, 18–19.

Norman A (1980) *Rights and Risks. A Discussion Document on Civil Liberty in Old Age*. London: Centre for Policy on Ageing.

Norman A (1987) Risk or restraint. *Nursing Times* 83(30).

Ogg J and Bennett G (1992) Elder Abuse in Britain. *British Medical Journal* 305: 998–99.

Pillener K (1993) *International Symposium on Elder Abuse*. Unpublished conference notes, Stoke-on-Trent.

Public Trust Office (1994) *Enduring Powers of Attorney*. London: Public Trust Office.

Ramprogus V and Gibson J (1991) Assessing restraints. *Nursing Times* 87(26): 45–47.

Reiser S J, Bursztajn H J, Appelbaum P S and Gutheil T G (1987) *Divided Staffs, Divided Selves. A Case Approach to Mental Health Ethics*. Cambridge: Cambridge University Press.

Royal College of Nursing (1992) *Focus on Restraint*, 2nd edn. London: Scutari Press.

Rumbold G (1989) *Ethics in Nursing Practice*. London: Baillière Tindall.

Sadler C (1989) Driven to desperation. *Nursing Times* 85(27): 18–19.

Seedhouse D (1988) *Ethics. The Heart of Health Care*. London: John Wiley.

Sutton C (1992) *Confronting Elder Abuse*. London: HMSO, Social Service Inspectorate.

Tomlinson D (1993) *No Longer Afraid. The Safeguard of Older People in Domestic Settings*. London: HMSO.

Tschudin V (1986) *Ethics in Nursing*. London: Heinemann.

United Kingdom Central Council (1992) *Code of Professional Conduct*, 3rd edn. London: UKCC.

Wolf R (1993) *International Symposium on Elder Abuse*. Unpublished conference notes, Stoke-on-Trent.

Wynne Harley D (1991) *Living Dangerously: Risk Taking, Safety and Older People*. London: Counsel and Care.

Yeo M (ed.) (1991) *Concepts and Cases in Nursing Ethics*. Ontario: Broadview Press.

9 Managing Change
Implementing new practice

'Nobody likes change'. This statement may be a cliché but demonstrates how most people feel about change. Equally, some professionals are heard to express the view that they are 'always changing' and that it's nothing new. Whatever the truth of these two statements a shift in the organisational structure or culture of the unit will have a dramatic effect on a group of staff. There are different types of change, some being easier to accept than others. Some changes may simply equate to 'tinkering around the edges of a job or activity', such as changing the forms that are filled in or rescheduling a meeting to make it more convenient for staff. Another change, familiar to professionals who work in statutory organisations, is the abrupt role or function change that occurs when reorganisation is implemented. This type of change, which is hard to cope with, is usually sharp and abrupt and the professional will find themselves in a new role virtually overnight.

The most difficult type of change for staff to tolerate is where the lead professional or manager recognises that extensive changes need to occur in order to improve an aspect or aspects of care delivery. This type of change will challenge the very heart of an organisation's culture and belief system and, because of this, may possibly provoke considerable resistance during the change process.

Where a staff group intends to promote a positive approach to caring for people with dementia it is likely that they will be involved in implementing a number of changes as they become more aware of the needs of the service users. It is important that care professionals investigate and understand some change theories and how they affect practice in order to offer a better quality of care to the client group, and to enable staff to experience a more satisfying professional role within the organisation. To implement successfully any of the practices that have been suggested in this book will require clear vision, planning, understanding and tenacity on the part of the change implementer. It will involve risk, yet if successful the reward for both client and professional can be substantial.

POINTS TO PONDER

- Do you ever think to yourself that you ought to start taking some exercise or go on a diet, but never do anything about it?

- Would you be more likely to have taken action if you had been told by your GP that you would not obtain life insurance if you did not take more exercise or lose weight?

- Think back over your career in the caring profession. Is there a practice that you used to do without question, which you now know is bad practice?

- Have you ever had to start doing something differently against your better judgement, only to subsequently realise that the change was a good idea?

- Can you identify among your colleagues who would resist change; do you know why?

- Are you ever given the opportunity in your team to share what aspirations you have for your unit?

- Who holds the most power in your service: is it the manager or someone else?

- Do you know why particular care practices have developed in your place of work? Who instigated them?

FACTORS THAT AFFECT CHANGE

A care professional may have a dream of how care could be improved or how innovative practice could be put into place. Having the vision is one thing, but the problems involved in helping other staff to share that vision can be immense, for some people do not have the ability to see how a change in practice will improve life, but can only see how the change will destroy or upset what they know and value as familiar. Change involves breaking up old patterns of work, of attitude and belief and building new ones (Owen 1985). It is important that there is congruence between the beliefs underlying practice and the practice itself. There will be tension if the inner beliefs of the care professionals remain at odds with the new philosophy of care. The need to break down and then rebuild a unit's philosophy will generate insecurity and pose a threat that may generate aggressive responses from the staff team as they try to protect themselves individually or as a group from the 'predator'.

FORMS OF MOTION AND CHANGE

Different levels of change occur within organisations, but all affect the day to day care of the older person. Moss Kanter, Steen and Jick (1992) identified three main areas of movement within the total organisation. First, there is the movement of the total organisation as it relates to the environment; within care settings this might relate to the relationship of Health Authorities to Social Services. Second, the movement of one specific unit or department within an organisation in relation to another; thirdly, the movement that occurs within staff teams. This can happen when there are changes in personnel and staff may be manoeuvring for power or status. Events that appear quite removed from the direct care setting may have a consequence on that unit, both in the short- and long-term.

Within these areas of movement there are three ways in which change may be manifested (Moss Kanter et al 1992). There is the 'identity change', where organisations have to change in relation to others, perhaps they become a supplier of a different 'product', or receive their funding from a different source. This identity change is most dramatically illustrated in the transformation of NHS directly supported units to NHS trust status, or the diversification of residential care settings into domiciliary care provision.

There are 'coordination changes' where the roles of personnel within the unit or organisation have to change. This may happen where departments are restructuring and taking the opportunity of reviewing and reprofiling the staffing component.

The third type of change is where there are changes in control. Moss Kanter et al (1992) identified this as usually reflecting power struggles between personalities within a team, or the team itself rising up against threatened change from an external force.

Any of these changes will affect staff; the way that change is experienced will often depend on the person's position in the organisation. For the organisation's executives or senior managers the change is often strategic. There will be an overview or broad policy statement that has an effect on the direction in which the organisation may go. This strategic development will usually be turned into an operational policy which will directly affect the middle managers, whose role will be to implement the change prescribed. Middle managers can be classified as the change implementers and senior managers will be change strategists. Where the change process is being conceived within a small unit the change implementer might well also be the change strategist.

Obviously, the main resource in care organisations is staff. This means that the impact of change on people cannot be ignored. The staff group often feel powerless to influence the change that is occurring, they may have difficulty in understanding the wider issues that are causing the change or may be being 'kept in the dark' about the rationale for the change by their managers. In reality, the staff group are far from powerless, they can choose to work with the change implementer or can resist the attempts to introduce change. A common response to this perceived powerlessness is to attempt to increase their own power by joining forces into a formal or semi-formal group.

THE TYPE OF ORGANISATION

When considering an extensive change programme it is vital that the change implementer has taken account of the characteristics of the unit. Many factors influence the success or failure of a change strategy, and frequently some may only become obvious when staff are analysing the reason for the failure.

When a successful change has occurred in a unit it is often felt to be due to the influence of a dynamic innovative person. Similarly, when a change fails one or more members of staff are often seen to be responsible. Glenn and Richards (1977) describe 'make or break' personnel who have a pivotal role in any change programme, yet more recent studies have established an interesting theory that sees the environment as the most influential factor in the implementation of change (Milne 1985). It is difficult to see how an environment that will facilitate change will be achieved without a dedicated and charismatic innovator leading the way. It is probable that the most successful changes occur where there is someone who is keen to improve their care practice and a positive environment where change can take place.

The environment most likely to embrace change is the 'learning organisation'; this kind of organisation will be diametrically opposed to the closed organisation that creates a 'sweep it under the carpet' school of management (Carle 1993). This type of organisation may sound familiar to some people; if you make a mistake you cover it up, hoping that no one else will find out while you sit tight until the heat is off! If the mistake is subsequently discovered you blame someone else. The learning organisation is more open and more positive. In essence, if a mistake occurs it is owned and the consequences are assessed, the incident is reported immediately and the reasons for it occurring are investigated. If there is a flaw in the process it is rectified, in order to prevent a recurrence. Apocryphal stories are told about Japanese business people being amused that their English counterparts' response to a problem is to think of a solution, whereas the Japanese will look for a cause.

CREATING A LEARNING ORGANISATION

The learning organisation has been analysed in great depth by Senge (1990) who identifies five components to the the learning organisation.

Personal Mastery

A more familiar term would probably be 'personal development'; individuals should have opportunities to develop their personal vision and to reflect on their contribution to the unit or team. The individual should be encouraged to develop an understanding of their own needs and those of their colleagues. They should see team members as interdependent, with each member being able to influence events. People should also be encouraged to question and should have managers who will listen positively and consider the suggestions made.

Shared Vision

The team should have a shared long-term vision. In an ideal situation all team members will share the vision; in reality people will be at different stages of understanding and realisation. The team will need to be assisted in this by the provision of appropriate information from the managers, both about their own unit and about wider organisational issues. It is important that a team sees how they fit into the total picture of a service or organisation and how the organisation is affected by external factors.

Team Learning

A good team will have evolved a strategy for decision-making and conflict resolution. It will have learned to be an effective team where each member is valued for what they bring to the unit. Senge (1990) describes the process of team learning as also needing to include the development of clear avenues of communication and formulating ways of ensuring that projects are not sabotaged by powerful group members.

Mental Models

The environment must be developed in such a way that people's basic assumptions can be challenged supportively. The team should be encouraged to describe its value base, to examine their behaviour and assess if there is congruence between their beliefs and their practice. For some units and individuals this will be a new experience and the managers of the unit may need to give 'permission' for staff to spend time talking about apparently abstract ideas and give positive messages that comments, questions and constructive criticism of the service are welcomed.

Systems Thinking

The last category Senge (1990) highlights is one of integration and cohesiveness, where all the other four categories must come to work together in order to create the learning environment. It is important to appreciate that a 'learning organisation' cannot be created overnight; the usual estimate of the time taken to turn around an organisation is 5 years. It is important not to give up too soon. There will be setbacks and times when other issues take precedence. The team needs to remember that what they are trying to achieve is a total change in the way work is viewed, a change in attitude and openness. Staff will need to be reminded of the objectives of the exercise and be assisted to see how the elements fit together. Carle (1993) quotes two examples that typify changing an organisation:

> The harder you push, the harder the system pulls back

and

> Dividing an elephant in half does not produce two small elephants.

POWER

It is important, when planning major change, that the understanding of the culture of the organisation and unit includes an analysis of where the power lies. The power held by the change agent can be used in a variety of ways and can take many forms. There are a variety of bases for power (Sullivan and Decker 1988) and each lends itself to different uses. The most obvious kind of power base is 'legitimate' power, where the change agent is also the manager. In this situation staff will feel obliged to do what is required of them because of their subordinate position.

Where the change agent is in an advisory capacity and has no management control, they may have to rely on 'expert' power. Expert power develops over time and is based on the knowledge and expertise that the person has to offer. This type of power often means that the change agent has to argue change through a purely knowledge-based perspective and will have no authority to fall back on. For this situation to be successful the change agent will need to have the clear and unambiguous support of the managers of the unit.

Information and knowledge about an organisation can give power. Occasionally, perhaps through work on a committee or through a trade union, a member of staff may have more information about the organisation and plans than the manager. This information may be used within a team to resist changes and 'fend off' the change agent. Managers often use the 'knowledge is power' principle as a conscious ploy in order to keep control over a situation. Good communication requires that staff are made aware of those issues that will help them understand the environment in which they work. All members of staff do not need to know everything, but managers need to have clear criteria for deciding what they share with staff members and for ensuring that staff in similar positions are told the same information.

The least popular power base is 'coercive power', which is often based on the negative aspects of someone's performance. It is used by some managers out of necessity and for some it only reinforces the hierarchy.

Within any institutional setting the use of power in any of these forms will change throughout the day and will depend on the activities and interactions occurring. People receiving services can also use power to obtain information (Roth 1984). It must be borne in mind that some people with dementia will not have lost their communication skills and may be 'in control' of their care and hold the power base.

When identifying the power base within a professional team, it is important to analyse the positions of all the personnel, the power they may have and what form it might take. Unqualified staff are likely to be just as powerful as qualified staff. This may happen because there are more unqualified staff in the unit, or because of their position in offering the majority of the direct care. They can use the power of knowledge when discussing clients and be selective with information to the person in charge, even to the most senior members of the team if they choose (Strauss et al 1963).

The negotiated order of power is an integral part of an organisation and does not necessarily follow the most obvious path. The change agent should not only identify the hierarchy of structural power, but also clarify who holds the group power. They will need to be aware that power is not necessarily about conflict (Hamson et al 1992). The power of knowledge can be used as a positive force but may intimidate some staff, reinforcing 'what they do not know'. If knowledge power is used productively by the change agent it should be associated with a sound communication strategy and a commitment to reinforce positively the existing skills and current good practice of the group.

CULTURE

It is clearly recognised and accepted that each country or ethnic group has its own culture; equally, each organisation will have its own culture. A culture is developed over generations and is a system of beliefs, language and activity that are unique to a certain group. Cultures can be cultivated by senior managers in an effort to create the desired environment. This can be done by producing mission statements, corporate logos and specific presentation methods; for example, uniforms and name badges.

The other more covert culture is the inner culture; the way a unit works together, the unwritten rules and the basic assumptions of the staff group. There have been a number of theories produced on organisational culture, but the one that has proved particularly popular in the United Kingdom is Charles Handy's theory (1986). He identified four different types of cultures that exist, but emphasises that different cultures are suited to different kinds of organisations and it is not possible to define one type as always preferable. Specific behaviour patterns are required in different situations and the 'right' culture might only be achieved if it is taken in relation to other factors. An appraisal of these four cultures identifies them as the *power culture*, which is characterised by a strong charismatic person who is the central leader. It is personality-based and the team centres around the leader. It is a good culture for speed and decision-making. The *role culture* is rather more predictable and encompasses a team that is efficient when life is predictable. New innovations, when accepted, work alongside entrenched practice and not across it. It is rather hierarchical and does not cope easily with change. By contrast, *task culture* is a team activity that bases its performance on results. It is a creative culture that relies upon expertise and not on positional authority. If there is a positive environment this type of culture will be very successful. The fourth organisational culture outlined by

Handy (1986) is the *person culture*, where the 'team' is, in reality, a group of professionals who happen to work together. Their philosophy is that the organisation is there to help the individual and management is a chore. Local myths and rituals are built up around the idiosyncrasies of these personalities (Hamson et al 1992). It is quite feasible to have a number of different cultures in a large organisation, each one overlapping. Many staff will have had the experience of working in different departments of the same organisation, each department expected by senior managers to work to the same basic principles, but there will be a world of difference in how the departments operate and how they feel both to the staff member and to the service user.

When considering how to create an environment where change has the greatest opportunity to take place it is important to identify which culture is the most desirable one to aim towards. The power base will also influence how successful a culture will be. Hamson et al (1992) identify the location of the dominant power in each ideal culture type, as follows.

Power culture: power held by key individuals at the centre of the web.

Role culture: power and authority are largely coterminous. Expert power is accepted as 'on tap but not on top'.

Task culture: power is widely dispersed, skills of all experts are valued.

Person culture: power lies with the star individuals and is dictatorial in nature.

RESISTANCE TO CHANGE

One of the most useful areas to be aware of in the management of change is that of the resistance that different staff may present. Relationships within a staff group can develop and affect how the team interacts with each other and with the change implementer. It might only become apparent how resistant a staff group is to change when they are actually put in the position of having to change their practice or attitudes (Schon 1970). Schon describes fundamental resistance to change as 'dynamic conservatism' where staff fight relentlessly to remain the same. The individual or the group can, in becoming dynamic in their resistance to change, lose sight of why they are resisting change. In some staff groups each member resisting change may be doing so for different reasons, it may be an unconscious activity or a conscious conspiracy and the energy expended can be as great as is required to effect the original change requirement.

A traditional simplistic analogy about change is that of an ice cube. It requires energy to keep it frozen and energy to make it melt. Once it melts to the fluid state and the change has occurred it can be refrozen into a different shape. Interestingly, it takes much less energy to keep an ice cube frozen than it takes to melt it. Of course, ice does not have the complication of containing human emotion!

The response to change for some staff may be similar to a bereavement: they are mourning the loss of their stable state. In bereavement the person experiences denial, anger and sadness. Even if the change is accepted in principle staff may still need to pass through these stages (Weil 1991).

SOME EXAMPLES OF RESISTANCE

Where the change agent is seeking to convince others that there is a need to change they can feel lonely, isolated and in need of some support. The feelings of isolation can at times be overwhelming (Wright 1985). Resistance may at first be quite gentle in terms of conversations or meetings where there is some disagreement. However, the more persistent the change agent, the more resistant the change resister may become. Their determination to preserve the status quo may cause them to make attacks on the change agent's evidence, and if that does not have an effect they may resort to attempts to undermine the agent on personal grounds, perhaps by trying to discredit them. Quite often a few strong personalities will join forces and present a cohesive group in their fight against change. The change agent's attempts to reason with more open-minded members of the team may be overshadowed by this group. If there is evidence of this it may be appropriate to confront the group in a way which would establish the way forward for the whole team. This action might involve a small but symbolic presentation, perhaps instructing some specific activity: for example, removing a piece of furniture, sending someone on a training course or changing someone's shift, but it is vital that the change agent is clear in their mind what the end result is going to be. If the change that has to be effected is important enough, the staff who are demonstrating the most active dynamic conservatism may have to leave the unit, either by their own choice or as a decision of the manager. This could, in some situations, be the only way forward and the change agent must understand and try to accept that, if the changes being implemented are for the greater good, it may be acceptable to have some casualties.

Now that the market economy has entered the world of health and social care it is important that staff at all levels are aware that no one person is indispensable. It is important for staff to have the opportunity to learn to change and adapt in ways that will cause them the least amount of pain and suffering. Even in the most positive environment there are sometimes difficulties and conflict which result in a flashpoint of change, where the old order is overwhelmed and new patterns appear and reinforce each other in a better integrated system (Owen 1983).

The change agent must hold on to their dream. It is vital that they are aware of their own behaviour, their status and other situations around them and, however many times the change agent is beaten back or blown off course, they should continue to work towards that objective. The role of change agent is an isolated one but has, finally, great professional rewards if the person can hold on (Plant 1987).

IMPLEMENTING CHANGE

Having examined some of the theory of change, the rest of this chapter will consider the practical issues associated with the successful implementation of change.

Hopefully, the material in the first eight chapters of this book will have provided a number of pointers to the ways in which services can be altered to provide a higher quality experience for people with dementia. Any change needs to be carefully considered and planned; successful changes clearly do not simply 'happen'. The processes involved in implementing change can be broken down into four broad steps: deciding, planning, implementing and monitoring. Within each of these categories there are several factors to be considered. It is normal to have to invest more time and effort on the 'deciding and planning' stages than on the actual implementation.

Deciding

It may be that several things need to be changed. The first stage of decision-making must be to assess which change to try to institute first.

What change to make first

This may sound like a simple question but it is necessary to give consideration to which change should come first. Is it better to tackle some major issue or 'tinker' with a less important matter? The crucial criteria that should be considered include an estimation of the likelihood of successfully achieving the desired outcome. If the first attempt to alter the service fails staff and managers may not be willing to try again and the process and the change agent will have lost credibility.

The decision should also include a judgement about which change will result in a noticeable gain for service users and staff. If a change is achieved, but few people notice the difference, the effort, time and resources put into the change process may be deemed to have been wasted. The gain may take one of several forms; it may be a better service, more service, less waste, a quicker response, more flexibility, more job satisfaction or improved 'value for money'.

Some changes will involve the commitment of additional resources, perhaps in terms of more staff or more equipment. Other changes will not require this additional investment. It must not be assumed that all important changes automatically involve more money; this can lead teams to avoiding even considering making changes on the basis that the necessary budgets will never be available. Important improvements in the quality of service offered can be made by the changing of staff attitudes, yet this, although hard to achieve, does not involve additional finances. Where the planned change does require additional resources it is important to be as accurate as possible in the estimates of what will be required. There is a tendency to underestimate expense in order to make the scheme seem more attractive. The danger is that overspending may result in the successful implementation of change being tainted by claims of extravagance and any subsequent plans being rejected.

In making the decision about which change should be made first you must try to ensure that a single issue change has been selected. It is important to concentrate on one thing at a time; if you try to change several things at once the confusion is distressing to both residents and staff and if you encounter problems there is little chance of analysing what and how it went wrong. An example could be recognition that the food served on a unit is inappropriate. A decision is made to introduce a choice of main meal each lunchtime and offer a cooked high tea each evening. After a week of this new order the chef reports that the kitchen staff cannot cope. It will be difficult to find out if the main factor leading to this has been the need to prepare an alternative main course or the teatime dish. It would have been preferable to introduce one of these changes at a time, but to have a clear idea of the final desired position. The second change would only be introduced when the first change had been implemented to an agreed standard.

Defining the change

A decision has been made about the need to change and about what change to make first. Professional care staff responsible for implementing change need to be clear about the change and its intended aims and goals. The more clearly these can be defined at the outset the easier it will be to assess how well the change has been achieved. The aims and goals will form the 'performance indicators' when the change is being monitored.

It may be decided that the required change is to improve the way incontinence is managed in the unit. While this is a laudable aim there needs to be much more clarity about what this actually means. Imagine what might happen if this is the only information a staff group is given. Some staff could decide that they should consider the introduction of a more effective system for assessing incontinence; another group may decide that it means they should regularly toilet everyone every hour rather than every 2 hours. Yet another group of staff could try to achieve the desired change by insisting that everyone is 'padded up'.

The definition of the change being introduced should include some explanation about 'how' it will be achieved and must be backed by a clear idea of what will indicate whether the change has been achieved or not. In the example above, where staff try to achieve an improvement in continence, the key indicators could include both a decrease and an increase in the use of incontinence equipment. Clarification of the objectives of the change and the methods to be used to achieve it will usually lead to more appropriate and relevant indicators becoming obvious.

Why change?

Successful change relies not only on clarity about the change itself but also about the reason for changing. The most common reason for introducing a change is dissatisfaction with a current situation and a desire to improve things. It is important that the staff group can agree on a starting point. There needs to be a consensus on 'where are we now?' and, if possible, broad agreement about the need to do things differently. It should be possible for the staff group to describe the desired end point in answer to the question 'where do we want to be?' It is often helpful for a staff group to agree and produce a written description of the organisation or service as it will be after the change has happened. In any organisation there will be a number of reasons why some professionals think change is a good idea. Most care professionals will be interested in changes that improve the quality of the service without making their jobs more difficult, dangerous or complicated. The people who manage the unit or service will want to improve the service to the user but will also be concerned with its 'marketability' and its cost. There will be other people in the organisation who have special interests such as 'health and safety' or 'equal opportunities'; the person leading the change must take account of all of these aspects and be able to convince each person in the organisation of the merits of the change. This may involve the change agent in being able to describe the benefits of change in a variety of ways.

When to make the change

The person responsible for introducing the change will want to consider when to introduce the process. The timing should reflect sensitivity to other pressures on the service; in its simplest form this may mean avoiding the summer holiday season or the period around Christmas. It may need to relate to the presence or absence of key members of staff and to the availability of money; it may be that any additional funding is easier to access at the beginning of the financial year or that there is a predicted underspend available in March that can be used. The plan for change may need to be prepared for consideration by other parts of the organisation or be submitted for scrutiny to a variety of committees. All these aspects must be taken into account and incorporated into the plan in order to optimise the chances of success. There will be times when changes have to happen, regardless of the appropriateness of the timing; equally, there are occasions when a 'window of opportunity' presents itself and should be taken advantage of.

Planning the change

This part of the process focuses on ways of ensuring that the planned change has the maximum support of managers, staff and other key personnel. These aspects can be thought of as equivalent to 'selling the idea'. During this stage it will be necessary to decide what to do if you only achieve partial support, if people wish to negotiate about the extent of the changes proposed, or the time scale for implementation. Where the plans include discussions with senior managers it may have been necessary to have a negotiating position and to have been prepared to compromise on the speed and scale of the implementation. The opening proposal during negotiation may have been to give all staff some specific training in communication skills within the next 6 months. The outcome of discussions may be to give half the staff some training within the next year with a commitment to review the position. It is never advisable to enter a negotiating position without being clear about what will constitute an acceptable minimum agreement.

Deciding who are the key players

When a change is being planned it is important for the person responsible for implementation to have some idea about who the important and influential people are who can either assist or resist the process. 'Stake holder analysis' can help to clarify the situation. Stake holders are those people who have an interest or who are involved in an organisation. They can be arranged in a matrix, depending on the power and the interest they have. Some people will be extremely interested in what happens but have little power, others will have power but little interest. The critically important people to consult and convince of the need for change are those players who have both power and interest. The results of this kind of analysis can be surprising, demonstrating that in some situations the key players are not the managers of the service but the finance officer and the trade union representative.

Predicting the obstacles

Any change is likely to cause resistance; most people find change unsettling and will fight to defend the status quo. Anyone wanting to implement change should have considered the probable obstacles that will be put in the way. Take, for instance, the case of a respite unit that, because of the nature of the service, has several admissions every week. It is part of the tradition of the unit that when staff are making up beds they automatically put 'inco' sheets on the bed. If the change agent decides that it would be better for this practice to alter they must consider the possible objections. In this particular situation it is highly probable that the objections will centre around the increased probability of soaking wet beds. The change agent will find it helpful to have some idea of what proportion of people admitted are incontinent at night and an explanation ready for staff about the impact of unnecessary incontinence equipment on older people. They may need to check that the mattresses all have waterproof covers and be clear that they are aware of the care practices of the night staff.

Force field analysis is one way of looking systematically at the pressures that will assist or hinder change (Lewin 1951). Force field analysis assumes that situations are in temporary equilibrium, with the forces acting to change the situation balanced by the forces acting to resist the change. If such forces can be identified it becomes possible to consider ways of changing their direction or strength. The technique involves recognising those factors that will assist a change to happen and those that will resist. It allows for a consideration of whether there is an opportunity to remove some of the resisting forces or whether the helpful forces can be added to or strengthened.

Planning the style of the change

Most people prefer to avoid confrontation wherever possible; when changes are being planned in a service, most managers will prefer to achieve the change with the support and cooperation of the staff group. In most service organisations this means that changes have been introduced incrementally. In the commercial and industrial sectors this has not always been the case. Sometimes the only way of keeping a business successful is to bring about dramatic changes over a short period of time. It has been demonstrated that in these situations there is a time and place for 'coercive or directive change' (Stace and Dunphy 1991). It has been shown that top performing companies have a range of approaches and use them appropriately as circumstances dictate. There is a lesson in this for people involved in care services, particularly given the exposure of most services to the market forces of a mixed economy. There will be times when achieving change through collaboration and cooperation will take too long and will be inappropriate. Equally, there will be changes that are so important to achieve that it becomes necessary to implement a 'dictatorial transformation'. In other words, the agent of change will say, 'you may not agree with the proposal but it is so important to the survival of the service that you will do as I say'.

It is important that the staff member responsible for introducing changes is clear about how this will be executed. Imagine the situation where a new manager takes over a unit providing residential care to older people with dementia. The new manager finds that staff morale is low and care practices poor. They also discover that there has been no staff meeting for more than 2 years. The manager takes the decision to reinstate staff meetings and sends out a note to staff suggesting that they consider when would be the best time to hold the meeting. The manager has no response to the notes and decides to put a poster containing the same message on the staff notice board. The poster is ignored and the manager finally decides that the staff are not interested in a staff meeting and abandons plans to introduce a change. It would have been more appropriate to tell the staff that there would be a meeting and that attendance was compulsory.

The agent of change and their role

Most programmes of change work best when someone is clearly identified as the driving force. As previously discussed, this role is not often comfortable; when change is suggested people usually recall what is good about the current situation.

In many staff groups initial discussion of change will be met with lack of interest; as discussions proceed there will be a growth in resistance and in negative emotions. Many of these emotions will be directed at the 'agent of change'. This person will need to take comfort from the fact that the very existence of negative feelings means that the staff group have begun to accept the inevitability of change.

The agent of change does not have to be the most senior person in the organisation, but they will usually need their support and commitment to invest resources in the programme of change. The agent of change must be the person with the vision and must ensure that they develop efficient and effective ways of communicating with all of the stake holders. This communication system must include ways of collecting comments and feedback as well as ways of disseminating information (Salaman 1992).

The successful agent of change will be able to demonstrate coherence between what needs to be done and how they plan to do it, they will have a sound plan based on a realistic assessment of internal and external factors and they will have a clear idea of the goal that they can explain convincingly to colleagues. They will also be able to underpin the change with a recognised theory. They will be convinced of the need for change and sure of success but they will have a range of alternative options should things begin to go wrong. They will have thought through the impact on all the people involved and be clear about the resources needed (Johnson and Scholes 1993).

Implementing the Change

There comes a time when all the decision-making and planning is completed and it is judged to be the best time to implement the planned change. Even where the planning has been faultless there is a need for a degree of flexibility. The plan may need to change as staff begin to bring it into operation; there will need to be a balance between making alterations to achieve the best result and sticking with the original concept in order to give the plan a real chance. During the period of implementation the person leading the change will need to be visible and available, both to provide information and to reinforce the required practice. The staff team may need reassurance and support and may need reminding about the rationale behind the change.

Monitoring Change

If the desired change was clearly described at the outset it should be possible to decide fairly easily if it has been achieved. In most cases there will not be constant or total compliance with the new way of doing things. Some staff will 'forget', others will continue to try to jeopardise the change and others may have misunderstood what was required. It is important that the person leading the change is able to reinforce positively good practice and be aware of the situations that cause the old ways to be used. It may be that the new practice is always used by staff of one shift and not another, or that staff forget the new practices when pressurised. There will need to be an analysis of how this can be improved; perhaps some staff need to work on different shifts with other colleagues to see the benefits of change or something needs to be done to change the pressure on the unit. There may be ways of demonstrating that the new way is quicker or easier, so that it becomes the preferred option when the service is fully stretched.

An example of this could be the use of new technology in a unit. On an imaginary assessment unit each discharge letter is handwritten by a member of staff. It is decided to introduce a lap-top computer with a standard discharge letter already prepared on it. Obviously, until staff are familiar with the system it will take longer, but with practice the process can take much less time and the letter will be easier to read.

If the planned change did not succeed it will be necessary to examine carefully what went wrong. There may be a single factor or a multitude of issues that 'got in the way'. Once these factors have been examined the decision can be taken about trying again or substantially changing the approach.

The last few years have seen immense changes in the way services for people with dementia are provided; the next decade will see a substantial increase in the number of people with dementia and it is probable that services will have to diversify and be responsive to an ever-changing situation. A successful unit or service will seek to try to be a 'learning organisation' where the process of change and development is continual and where change is welcomed by staff as a sign of health and vitality. Services must become proactive and perhaps there is merit in looking not at 'implementing changes' so much as 'continual development'.

ACTION FOR CHANGE

1. Make the decision to change something in your personal life, perhaps giving up smoking, getting fit or losing weight. Plan the change using the suggested steps in this chapter.

2. Implement the change, keeping a diary of how, why and when things happened and how you felt about the process.

3. Analyse what factors contributed to the change succeeding or failing. Are the factors external and beyond your control, or do they reflect a personal weakness or difficulty?

4. Find out about ways of addressing these weaknesses, either through training, coaching or mentoring.

5. Reflect on whether the processes involved in the change that you have attempted are similar to or different from those involved in making changes in the workplace. What lessons have you learned from the experience that you can apply at work?

6. Find out about a change that a colleague is hoping to make at work that you can support. Become their ally and assist them in the process. Try to be as objective as possible about what happens and how you would have done things differently.

7. Decide on a change that you want to make and a date by which you hope to have undertaken it and do it.

REFERENCES

Carle N (1993) *The Learning Organisation: Making it Relevant*. London: King's Fund Centre.

Glenn R N and Richards D (1977) Assessing the potential of change in institutions. *Psychiatric Quarterly* **49**: 322–30.

Hamson S, Hunter D, Monson G and Pollitt C (1992) *Just Managing: Power and Culture in the NHS*. London: Macmillan.

Handy C (1986) *Understanding Organisations*, 3rd edn. Harmondsworth: Penguin.

Johnson G and Scholes K (1993) *Exploring Corporate Strategy*. London: Prentice Hall.

Lewin K (1951) *Field Theory in Social Science*. London: Harper.

Milne D (1985) The more things change the more they stay the same. Factors affecting the implementation of the Nursing Process. *Journal of Advanced Nursing* **10**(1): 39–45.

Moss Kanter R, Steen B and Jick T (1992) *The Challenge of Organisational Change*. London: Unwin.

Owen G (1983) The stress of change. *Nursing Times* **79**(4): 44–46.

Owen G (1985) Innovation in nursing — the role of higher education in relation to nursing practice. *Journal of Advanced Nursing* **10**: 179–85.

Plant R (1987) *Managing Change and Making It Stick.* London: Fontana/Collins.

Roth J A (1984) Staff, inmate bargaining tactics in long term institutions. *Sociology of Health Issues* **6**(2): 111–31.

Salaman G (ed.) (1992) *Human Resource Strategies.* London: Oxford University Press.

Schon D (1970) Dynamic conservatism. *The Listener* **84**(2174): 724–28.

Senge P (1990) *The Fifth Discipline, The Art of the Learning Organisation.* New York: Doubleday.

Stace D and Dunphy D (1991) Beyond traditional paternalistic and developmental approaches. *International Journal of Human Resource Management* **2**(3).

Strauss A, Schatzman L, Ehblich D, Bucher R and Sabshin M (1963) The hospital and its negotiated order. *The Hospital in Modern Society.* USA: The Free Press of Glencoe.

Sullivan E and Decker P (1988) *Effective Management in Nursing,* 2nd edn. New York: Addison–Wesley.

Weil S (1991) *Learning to Change.* London: Office of Public Management.

Wright S (1985) Change in nursing: the application of change theory to practice. *Nursing Practice* **2**(83): 85–91.

10 The Quest for Quality

Professional development and quality assurance

There is an image that any service that offers care to older people is static, unexciting and undemanding; that the people who choose to work with older people are 'taking the easy way out' and will be less motivated, less skilled and less qualified than their counterparts in other services (Chapman and Marshall 1993). Many people would argue that this has never been true, others may acknowledge that there is a grain of truth behind this stereotype. Whichever is true there is an increasing number of people who are coming to realise that the last decade has seen substantial changes in services for people with dementia and that recent legislative changes are presenting real challenges to these services. This chapter will examine some of these factors and consider their impact on the development of services, of teams and of individuals.

POINTS TO PONDER

- Do you know how many potential users of your service (i.e. people with dementia) are in your area?
- How do you know that your service is what people want?
- Can you list any changes that there have been in the demand for your service, in the last 2 years? Can you explain why they occurred?
- How many ways do you have of measuring the quality of the service that you offer?
- When you are shopping for a new piece of furniture how do you decide what is 'value for money'?
- Think about the last training course that you attended. Did you want to go or were you sent?
- Recall the last time you succeeded with a client when others had failed. Can you identify the reasons why you succeeded?

- Think about the teams you are part of. Are you clear about your role in each of them and would other team members agree with you?

THE NHS AND COMMUNITY CARE ACT

The implementation of the National Health Service and Community Care Act in April 1993 has had a dramatic impact on the care of older people and on the services designed to support them. Money spent previously by the Department of Social Security on the purchase of residential and nursing care for older people has been transferred to Social Services departments. These departments are required to spend 85 per cent of this transferred money in the independent sector and financial disincentives were established for any departments choosing to continue to provide residential care directly. The Act emphasised the need for people to be offered holistic assessments that would lead to a 'needs led' 'package of care' comprising services drawn from a 'mixed economy of care' (Griffiths 1988).

This major change has had a dramatic impact on all of the services providing care for older people. In very general terms, fewer older people are choosing to enter residential or nursing care and are preferring to remain in their own homes supported by community-based services. This has, in turn, led to a higher level of vacancies in some residential and nursing homes with some businesses finding themselves in financial difficulties.

In most parts of the country, establishments that are registered to provide care to people with dementia have, to a large extent, been protected from this drop in demand but the people with dementia entering care are substantially more impaired than was the case some years ago. It can be predicted that some registered residential homes currently registered for 'elderly people' will choose to change their re-register category for the care of people with dementia in order to secure financial viability. How many homes make the change will depend, to a large extent, on the amount of the additional financial payment made to this category of home and the additional registration requirements demanded.

Changes in legislation and demand are also having an impact on Local Authority and Health Authority provision. In some parts of the country, Local Authorities have shed most or all of their residential provision, in other areas they are concentrating their services on respite care and assessment. Most Health Authorities are also reducing the number of continuing care beds. People with dementia may have a terminal illness but few can look forward to 'free' continuing care.

Local Authorities are also required, by the NHS & Community Care Act, to publish 'eligibility' criteria that govern access to their services. This has forced departments to state clearly that there are some people who will be assessed as having few urgent needs and who will not be guaranteed a service. Only people in the higher bands of each set of criteria will be guaranteed a service; this has led many Social Services departments to an appreciation that older people with dementia will, in the future, form the largest proportion of 'eligible' service users.

Those older people who are choosing to stay at home with support are being offered 'packages of care' by Social Services staff following a holistic assessment. The 'package of care' may be made up of a mixture of services provided by the Social Services department and some purchased from the independent sector. As time passes staff arranging these packages and staff providing services have become more confident and entrepreneurial and a range of innovative services are beginning to be established to meet specific needs. These services may range from an individual meal purchased from the local public house to 'respite at home' and night sitting.

The Local Authorities are expected to show a clear distinction between 'purchasing' and 'provider' roles, similar to that required of the Health Service some years ago. This reorganisation has forced these agencies to become more 'businesslike', paying increasing attention to unit costs, 'value for money', market share and rationalisation. Similarly, independent sector providers are expected to be able to tender for services, understanding and complying with service specifications and contract conditions. Professional care staff, in any agency, need to develop appropriate 'business skills'. It is no longer enough to be simply interested in care. The survival of any service may depend on the manager's ability to market and package the service.

DEMOGRAPHY

There has been a substantial increase in the numbers of 'old old' people in the last decade (OPCS 1991). The incidence of dementia is directly proportional to age and rises rapidly in people aged 85 years and over; recent research indicates figures of 18.5 per cent in men and 22.8 per cent in women aged 85–89 years (Hofman, Roca and Brayne 1991). A consideration of the probable number of people with dementia in a particular location will indicate that even the most innovative service will only be in touch with a small proportion of potential users. It follows that any service will probably have to ration its services in some way. This requires the service to be clear about the way it allocates its resources and to be able to justify its decisions.

THE DEMENTIA CARE BUSINESS

The coming years will see pressure on existing services to develop and diversify. Apart from a need to find new ways of providing care there is a growing awareness that the quality of services needs to change. Alongside this is the pressure to be more 'businesslike'. Many care professionals will have shied away from this notion, believing that unit costs, throughputs and cost benefit analysis have little to do with quality care services. In reality, no service can guarantee its survival unless it can demonstrate that it provides 'value for money' and is what 'customers' want. Care professionals managing services need to be able to provide a range of services that are sensitive to the needs of older people with dementia and their carers, that is affordable, of an acceptable quality and attracts appropriate referrals. For example, it is unwise to operate a long-stay unit that struggles to maintain its occupancy if there is a desperate demand for respite care. Equally, it is not sensible to offer a high cost service with a plethora of 'luxury trimmings' if 90 per cent of your potential customers can be predicted to require financial support from the Local Authority. All services, no matter how well established or well thought of, must become market sensitive. Times are changing rapidly and only those facilities that are based on sound market research and sound business principles will survive. In the field of dementia care this may mean developing a particular style of service, providing new services, or providing a service for a particular kind of person, perhaps the younger person with dementia or the person with challenging behaviour.

PROFESSIONAL DEVELOPMENT

The care of people with dementia provides challenges for both health and social care agencies, being one of the most appropriate services for a joint or collaborative commissioning approach. In a number of areas of the country care services have been developed and are provided by joint health and social care teams.

The number of qualified care staff working with older people with dementia has been limited, but there are signs that things are changing in both health and social care settings, perhaps best demonstrated by the recent launch of the *Journal of Dementia Care*. There is a growing awareness that many of the techniques of social work are appropriate to working with people with dementia (Chapman and Marshall 1993). This process is being assisted by the formation, in many Social Services departments, of specialist 'adult' teams. These teams, led by specialist managers, are better able to focus on the needs of older people without being distracted by the pressures of child protection work. Within the sphere of nursing there is more emphasis on a 'therapeutic' approach and there have been acknowledgements in the associated fields of occupational therapy and physiotherapy that the care of older people with dementia is a speciality in its own right.

MONITORING QUALITY

In the last few years people involved in providing care have become interested in examining the quality of the services they provide; part of the business ethic has included a requirement to monitor and assure quality.

Earlier chapters of this book have attempted to show how quality care can be provided and how services can be changed and developed to provide a more appropriate style of service for people with dementia. Care professionals need to be aware that having established high quality care it needs to be carefully and thoroughly monitored; without systems of quality assurance in place the quality will invariably slip backwards.

In the 1990s the terms Quality and Quality Assurance, Audit, Protocols and Audit Tools have become as much a part of professional language as Assessment, Care Planning or Evaluation. The word 'quality' is, however, perhaps the word that has been used throughout the past two or three decades, but its usage and understanding has changed. In the 1960s 'quality' was a term used to reflect the best that was available, a quality item that was well made and would cost a fair price. Today the term 'quality' refers to a continuum rather than an end product (Norman and Redfern 1993). Attached to the term 'quality' are many other words that are often used inaccurately.

Quality management is the philosophy of leading an organisation into managing quality. *Quality control* is monitoring the product or the process. *Quality assurance* looks at the prevention of quality problems through planned systematic activities.

Quality assurance is an infinite cyclical process of activity which includes the identification of quality, the measuring of quality and the taking of action (Norman and Redfern 1993). There are a number of models that look at a framework for quality assurance: the most famous is probably that of Donabedian (1980), who describes the process as consisting of three interrelated components — structure, process and outcome. Lang's quality assurance process has an open circular movement, including setting standards, identifying present practice and using the difference to dictate a course of action (Koch 1992). The third model, possibly less well known by author but easily identifiable, is the Marker Umbrella Model (Marker 1987). This model insists on total staff commitment and emphasises systematic review of patient care, staff performance and the role of the organisation (Koch 1992).

Any one of these models, or indeed a combination of them, would fit into the philosophy of Total Quality Management (TQM). This style of quality assurance developed within industry and has grown out of the need to maintain competitiveness with improved quality. The principle of TQM encompasses the whole organisation, taking a corporate approach to issues of quality, to embrace the measurement of quality within everyone's work ethic and to have a continuous cycle of activity that assesses and takes action to improve standards. An organisation that embraces TQM has a wholehearted commitment to the service user and feels comfortable in looking continuously at practice and improving the quality of that service to the user. It is also important within the philosophy of TQM to be proactive and be prepared to consider improving service and care before a user complains about a specific aspect. It encompasses open communication at all levels, human resource development and customer feedback (McSweeney 1992).

Whichever model of quality assurance is used it always depends on a systematic approach which must ensure the following.

- Quality is seen as a responsibility of every staff member. It must become part of the culture of the service.

- Quality assurance must be part of 'normal' activity and not an occasional additional function that happens when there is nothing more urgent to attend to.

- All services, plans and policies must be focused on the people using the service and there must be mechanisms in place to ensure that people who use the service are involved in decisions about the service (Kitson 1989).

- The focus must be on preventing, rather than detecting, problems.

- Goals and targets (or performance indicators) for the service should be clearly stated and well publicised both within the staff group and among people who use the services.

• Complaints must be seen as a spur to improvement and a challenge rather than a nuisance or a threat.

There are three main steps to developing a quality control system. The first stage consists of an analysis which seeks to detail the tasks, structures, processes and outcomes that are involved in the service. This should ensure that any quality assurance system looks at all of the facets of the service.

The second stage is to devise a 'quality plan' and choose appropriate methods of audit. The final stage includes deciding on 'corrective actions'.

GETTING STARTED, ANALYSING THE SERVICE

Before looking at the whole service it is useful to examine the management systems that currently exist. This has the benefit of showing staff in the service that managers are willing to examine critically their own contributions to the service. Areas for inspection could include recruitment, training, the organisation of meetings, supervision and communication systems. This is the time for managers of services to be brave and ask the staff they manage to comment on the managers' skills and for managers to undertake self appraisal (Barlow 1990).

Analysing the service requires managers to be specific about all of the elements of service. The more detailed the description at this stage, the more likely that the quality plan will be comprehensive. The description should include all the tasks undertaken, all the resources used to provide the service, all the processes entailed and all the possible outputs and outcomes (Donabedian 1966). The beginning of an analysis of a 'respite at home' service may look like this:

Tasks	Resources	Processes	Outputs	Outcomes
To provide respite at home	Care workers Secretary Manager Transport Budget	Referral Assessment Allocation Reviewing Supervision	Hours per user No. of referrals Staff sickness Response time	Carers supported Quality of life improved Choice of service offered

DRAWING UP A QUALITY PLAN

The second step in the compilation of a quality assurance plan involves being clear about what information you need to know in order to assure quality, knowing what is already available and deciding on ways of collecting the data that is not currently collected. The manager of a 'respite at home' service may already be able to access information on budgets, travel costs, referral patterns and overtime payments but may decide that they need information on the following.

- The length of time someone waits between referral and a worker being allocated.
- The number of telephone enquiries the service deals with each week.
- The number of people enquiring about the service who subsequently choose not to use it.
- The amount of time it takes to process time sheets each week.
- The number of service users receiving one visit a week, two visits a week, etc.
- The number of reviews not completed on time.
- The satisfaction levels of carers using the service.

The manager must decide how this information is collected and who will be responsible; they also need to decide if the information will be collected occasionally (a snapshot) or continuously (ongoing). They also need to know how they are going to collate the data and who will have access to it. The manager also needs to be confident that the resources involved in the data collection can be justified.

The overall quality plan should list the areas of service to be covered, the measurement tools to be used and the frequency of the 'measurement'. As an example, the carer's view of the respite service could be measured by asking three carers to complete a standard questionnaire each month; the number of reviews not completed on time could be ascertained by asking each worker to log outstanding reviews every 3 months; the length of time taken to allocate a worker could become a standing item for discussion in the weekly staff meeting. The best quality plans include a range of tools and have fixed on a frequency of assurance that is appropriate to the service element. Some of the more common 'tools' would include 'inspections, quality circles, surveys, peer reviews, tracking, shadowing and audit'. Each tool has specific advantages and disadvantages and requires different levels of resourcing. 'Audit' has changed its meaning over the past three decades: it is now an accepted term meaning a measurement necessary to provide practitioners with information on whether improvement is required (Norman and Redfern 1993).

STANDARD SETTING

An integral part of Audit and Quality Assurance in care settings, both statutory and in the independent sector, is the preparation of written standards. These should identify what people can expect to find in the service and should be used as an indicator for improvement (Koch 1992). Standard setting is exacting, as it is vital that the language used is clear and easily understood and that the outcome is in some way measurable. The best standards are determined by a 'bottom up approach'; there is a danger that they will be seen as rather remote if set and imposed by the organisation. Within the market economy senior managers need standards and measurable outcome to assist in the promotion and marketing of their service. Commissioners and Purchasers find standards useful to assist in their inspection of the quality of service provision and the users should have open access to the unit standards in order to be able to measure the service they receive.

At the outset, most units or services will not have performance indicators unless they have been imposed on them by another part of the organisation. After the quality plan has been running for some months it will be possible to determine performance indicators that are specific to the service. In the example of 'overdue reviews', it may become obvious that there are usually 40 late reviews; it may be decided that if this became more of a priority for staff, the numbers could be reduced to 15 over a period of a year and that thereafter this should be the standard.

Most care professionals will only see the value of standards within the unit if they reflect the daily practice and the outcomes are neither too subjective to measure nor conversely simple head-counting exercises.

Any care professional wishing to implement a quality plan will have to acknowledge that many staff will find the process uncomfortable. They will need to be reassured that the objective of the exercise is to point out good practice and it should lead to efforts being targeted on those areas of work that need most attention. The focus of quality assurance work is the service and the processes that support it, not individual staff. It is important for the delivery of a high quality service that all the care professionals involved should have an understanding of the concept of standard setting, quality assurance and the principles of basic research (Koch 1992).

Quality assurance work usually involves collecting the views of service users; there will be times when it is difficult to ascertain the views of people with dementia, but this does not mean that staff should not always attempt to involve people. The discussions will take more time and the techniques will need to be adapted to suit individuals but it is possible to get a feeling for how people with dementia experience services. The views of advocates, family members and carers will be useful but are not a substitute for the views of the older person (NCVO 1991; Winn 1990).

A new technique has been developed during the last few years. Called Dementia Care Mapping (Kitwood and Bredin 1991), this technique allows trained observers to measure the quality of life of people with dementia in a systematic way. The tool is labour-intensive, requiring one observer to every six or seven older people and for the periods of observation to be extensive, perhaps 16–20 hours over several days. The benefit of the system is the wealth of data that is produced; it can be used to measure the quality of life for an individual, to measure the implementation of a care plan, to examine the differences between teams of staff and to examine changes in care over a period of time. When an establishment allows dementia care mapping to be used on its premises, staff will naturally experience some alarm at the prospect of being 'watched'. The novelty will soon wear off and the good news for staff is the possibility of being shown how small changes in staff behaviour can dramatically affect a person's quality of life.

Taking Corrective Action

All quality assurance work relies on information collection that must lead to action. The action may be something to help maintain current standards or to make changes to improve current practice. Sometimes the change will be within the sphere of control of the service manager, at other times it will need to be reported to a higher authority. There is no point in knowing where the weaknesses are in a service if the staff and managers of the service are unwilling to make changes!

Developing Teams

Undertaking quality assurance work in an attempt to maintain or improve services will always be easier if the staff involved in the service work together as an effective team. Teams do not simply happen. They need to be planned, developed and supported.

A team is taken usually to be a group of people who come together to carry out specific functions; the membership of the team may change and people may belong to more than one team at the same time. A community psychiatric nurse may belong to a locality team, a multidisciplinary team and be attached to a primary health care team. The basic assumption of a team is that the actions of one team member will impact on the others (Douglas, Ettridge and Fearnhead 1988).

Teams will vary in the way they are structured and the way they work; it takes effort and commitment from team members to make the team effective and efficient. The ability of a team to work well will take time to develop; members need to get to know one another, come to a common understanding of the team's purpose and be willing to agree on a way of working (Douglass 1992). Where a team, or part of a team, feels that it is dysfunctional remedial steps can be undertaken. These will include both team-building exercises and an analysis of the roles and functions of individuals within the team (Dyer 1987).

Team Building

Team building is not only appropriate when a new team is formed: it can be useful at any stage in a team's life. Working with people with dementia is a challenging occupation and places stresses on care professionals. Some of these stresses and pressures will be relieved if a team works well together and can offer support to its members. Occasionally this support may 'just happen', more usually it needs to be planned and designed. It is not indulgent for teams to take time out to look after themselves; teams in which members look after each other will nearly always be more effective. Traditionally, team building takes the form of an 'away day' for all staff involved in a unit or service. This can be almost impossible to arrange in many intensive services and team building will have to be built into other occasions, such as regular staff meetings. The exercises need to be carefully planned and consideration needs to be given to the use of a facilitator, the danger being that any staff member taking responsibility for organising team building can find their position on the outside of the team being reinforced.

Multidisciplinary Teams

Many teams providing care for people with dementia will contain members from a range of professional backgrounds. In these teams the senior medical member has usually become the leader, this position being explained in terms of 'clinical responsibility'. The most familiar example of this will be the psychogeriatrician with 'his team' of junior doctors, social workers, occupational therapists and nurses (Walton and McLachlan 1986). In this traditional model, the consultant is the leader and the decision-maker with other 'team members' being there to provide information or volunteer for work (or make the tea). This is not the only way such a team can operate; it can become more democratic and the decision-making can be shared. This is not to say that there ought not to be a chairperson. Most teams function best with someone 'organising' the meeting but the chairperson is not necessarily the most powerful person (Belbin 1981).

An effective multidisciplinary team needs to be based on mutual respect with each profession being valued for its special expertise and skill. It is often helpful for even the most stable and cooperative team to take time out occasionally from their tasks to re-examine the way they function, the roles team members take and the rules they operate by. These discussions can result in a team 'code of conduct' that may lay down rules concerning confidentiality, being listened to, decision-making and time-keeping.

Alongside the team-building programmes that have already been discussed there may be other activities that will enable a team to develop a closer working relationship and a mutual pride in quality care delivery. Within nursing organisations nursing development units (NDUs) have produced an ideal formula for improving the quality of care while developing the team and the profession. NDUs are specifically and explicitly committed to the development of nursing and nursing practice. Based in any care setting the units work towards innovative practices that can be evaluated and which have measurable outcomes (Wright 1989). The team has the opportunity to develop together and individually and takes the issue of change to improve the quality of care delivery as a fundamental part of the unit's philosophy (Wright 1989). This change can, however, sometimes be as hard to accept in an NDU as in any other care environment.

For care professionals who are not nurses practice development units (PDUs) (Williams and Lowry 1993) can offer the same opportunities to develop practice and improve quality using research-based methods. In PDUs the leader can be any professional who is clinically based. This leadership role for both types of unit is about facilitating, coordination, enabling and acting as a resource for team members. An integral part of the work activity is the forming and coordination of staff support groups. These groups may not have a direct impact on development and support (Milne, Walker and Bamford 1987), but may prove to be useful as a time to 'opt out' and take time to talk together about general unit issues.

DEVELOPMENT OF INDIVIDUAL SUPERVISION

Supervision has become an accepted method of supporting and developing staff in clinical situations. It has been an accepted feature of social work for many years and recently the Department of Health have stated that they consider it to be fundamental to safeguarding standards, development of professional expertise and the delivery of health care. It is accepted as a method of improving the quality of 'therapy' given as well as an important safety device for the client and the worker. There is still, however, some misconception that the only function of supervision is to allow the manager to scrutinise the work of the supervisee. This view, held by professionals, may reflect the methods of supervision used by the managers and the relationship between the manager and the supervisee.

It is generally accepted that the goals to supervision are threefold:

1. to expand the therapist's knowledge base;
2. to assist in developing clinical efficiency; and
3. to help develop autonomy and self esteem as a professional (Platt-Koch 1986).

It is also identified as a growth experience, enabling the interaction between supervisor and supervisee to be a method of counter transference of problems and learning blocks, thus allowing the supervisee to understand their reaction to the client (Ekstein and Wallerstein 1972).

Today's society demands control on care services, and supervision and staff support can offer a method of re-evaluating the service that is being offered, but more than that it offers the chance for staff to feel valued and to be able to express their worries and concerns about the nature of the work they are undertaking in a safe environment. The word 'supervisor' comes from the Latin *supervidere*, which means to look upon or survey (Rankin 1989), and this describes closely what supervision is. Staff need to be given the opportunity to sit back and reflect on the work they are doing and examine ways of improving care. They also need time to develop self-awareness and to consider some of the ethical and moral dilemmas involved in caring for people. For some staff the idea of clinical supervision can be very threatening, and some care professionals feel that if they work in a close environment they will automatically receive the support that is needed (Wilkin 1988). The value of this 'natural' kind of support is that it may not be appropriate to the needs of the worker or the service, in that it can be based on a sympathetic, rather than an empathetic, approach. Good supervision should always be positively constructive, but should not shy away from confrontation of the difficult or the sensitive.

DEALING WITH STRESS THROUGH SUPERVISION

The stress experienced by care professionals has attracted considerable attention from researchers over the last few years, particularly as stress is implicated increasingly as a cause of sickness, absenteeism, frustration and of staff leaving the caring professions. How people deal with stress varies enormously. The response to a situation depends on individual personality, physical make-up and past experience. Therefore, to emphasise stress as a universally unpleasant stimulus assumes that all individuals will respond similarly. This, of course, is not true and overwhelming stress for one person is motivating pressure for another. Stress needs to be dealt with on an individual basis; it is as important to meet the staff's individual needs as it is to meet the clients' (Copp 1988).

The relationship between different stresses and such effective states as distress, tension and dissatisfaction has been reported by a number of authors (e.g. Dewe 1989). Dewe looked at situations of stress and compiled a checklist of work stressors. The staff he interviewed indicated that their work generally left them feeling tense, with difficulty in 'switching off', tired and exhausted. A correlation was found between tiredness and tension. Dewe also identified that staff with different levels of responsibility, such as enrolled nurses and ward managers, identify different stressors and have different coping mechanisms.

It is important that individual and organisational resources are provided to allow people to deal with their own personal stress. This may be through the provision of supportive and positive structures through which staff can grow and develop. Dealing with stressful situations is also greatly assisted by good interpersonal relationships within the working environment.

Firth, McIntee and McKeown (1986) identified that respect, empathy and genuineness were important ingredients in a helping relationship that are particularly valued by staff.

APPROACHES TO SUPERVISION

Within the structure of supervision the allocation of the supervisor can be done in a number of ways. Within some services the supervisor is the line manager, within other situations a 'mentorship' system may be established. A mentor is said to be a guardian angel who watches over your career and guides you, modelling and shaping your professional development (Bracken and Davis 1989). However, the selection of the mentor is crucial. The mentor must be someone the member of staff respects and someone who can encourage and be aware of the supervisee's potential. Similarly, a traditional supervisory role will require mutual commitment for the relationship to work effectively.

Another development under the umbrella of supervision is the use of reflective practice. Reflection is the way in which a care professional can examine their practice and make sense of the issues that surround their actions. Supervision using reflection can help professionals unravel the complexities of caring (Johns and Butcher 1993). However, Darbyshire (1993) argues that reflective practice may simply be the latest trend in the caring profession. He argues that the very nature of nursing does not always allow for people to stand back from a situation and analyse all the alternatives. Within any caring profession there will be situations where action has to be taken based on intuitive knowledge, where any delay for debate may endanger the client. It is vital, however, that the professional in this situation is able to think about their actions afterwards and analyse and synthesise the incident. Environments must be created where open conversation can be held, to enable practitioners to reflect either in supervision, or within the team environment.

STAFF APPRAISAL

Developing a quality service for people with dementia must encompass continual staff appraisal and staff development. Caring for people is a dynamic process and the staff must be offered the opportunities to review themselves if they are to remain in touch with current thinking. Appraisal benefits not only the staff member; the employing organisation will also benefit from improved staff performance. The organisation must continually ensure that the service they provide is both of a high standard and is cost-effective; therefore any increase in effective practice and individual development will not only raise the quality of care given, but will enable the organisation to market their product more effectively.

The role of appraisal is seen to increase the contribution of individuals in their current job and to develop the potential abilities to meet the needs of the service in the future (Kerrane 1989). Accepted principles of appraisal revolve around supportive and constructive dialogue. The professional is often asked to analyse their own strengths and weaknesses before the interview and then present this analysis for discussion with their appraiser. An undisturbed interview in a private place encourages staff to identify what they can offer the service, what the service requires from them both now and in the future, and the interview should result in a mutually agreed development plan. Although many care professionals feel extremely anxious when introduced to the appraisal system this anxiety should be quickly dispelled if the session is handled by the manager as a learning experience (Herbert and Evans 1991). It is important for both parties to do the appropriate groundwork before going forward with the interview. The 'average' appraisal session can take up to 2 hours, with the possibility of additional time being committed subsequently by the appraiser as identified in the development plan. In an ideal world the development plans should be centred around personal and professional development; however, the market economy and purchaser/provider split dictates that the needs of the organisation must also be reflected (Herbert and Evans 1991). Appraisal systems encourage the development of professional autonomy, by involving staff in their own professional responsibilities to themselves, their clients and their organisation.

THE VALUE OF STAFF

For many professional groups the issue of the qualification and experience of staff working with people with dementia is high on the political agenda. For many years this area of health and social care has been considered as a 'non-speciality' where no particular skills are required as the clients need only 'basic care'. Training opportunities have traditionally been poor and geriatric services have been identified as dumping grounds for staff who were not good enough to work anywhere else. Thankfully, these images are slowly fading and the value of highly skilled and motivated care professionals working with older people is becoming recognised. The emergence of this speciality is, however, now facing the new threat of the internal market and the need for cost-effective services; consequently, particularly in Health Care establishments, skill mix and reprofiling reviews are being undertaken. Skill mix can be identified as the balance between trained and untrained, qualified and unqualified, supervisory and operative staff who work within a given service. The optimum skill mix is achieved when the desired standard of service is provided at the minimum cost which is consistent with the efficient deployment of staff (RCN 1992).

The crucial part of any skill mix review undertaken by service managers is the identification of tasks and the determining of the skills required. Within health care services there are a number of sophisticated packages for measuring the value and effect of the qualified nurse on patient outcome. *Criteria for Care* (Goldstone, Ball and Collier 1984), *Monitor* (Goldstone, Ball and Collier 1987) and *Senior Monitor* (Goldstone, Ball and

Collier 1988) are examples of these packages for general hospital settings which attempt to address complex issues. However, these packages have not addressed the complexity of caring for people with dementia.

Take the example of a senior manager in a hospital trust, who allocated to housekeepers the task of feeding the most dependent patients, as it was a 'menial task' and thus did not need to be undertaken by expensive qualified nurses. This scenario could easily be transferred to any social care setting or residential home. Some may argue that this senior manager was quite correct in his analysis and this was an appropriate cost-efficiency saving. Others, however, may disagree. Feeding patients involves a combination of skills and knowledge; people with dementia need particularly well trained staff who can establish a relationship, build trust and use skilful touch. The staff need to be able to understand both verbal and nonverbal communication and understand any physiological degeneration that may be occurring due to the dementia, or special dietary needs because of multiple pathology. Feeding patients is, therefore, not a mundane task!

Any efforts to review the skill mix in a setting should be accepted and treated as a potentially helpful process, although staff must ensure they have the ability to articulate and present the speciality they represent positively. In order to do this they need to be clear about the skills they use daily and be able to tease out the therapeutic content associated with basic caring tasks.

The problem for care professionals who undertake work with people with dementia is that much of the care has the appearance of being rather basic. The special quality of qualified care professionals is to blend knowledge, skill and experience into high quality care packages (Clark 1992).

THE VALUE OF THE UNQUALIFIED CARE WORKER

With the development of National Vocational Qualifications (NVQs) opportunities are now becoming available to people who may have a wealth of experience but who have not had the opportunity to formalise their training. With changing demography it is also evident that there will be fewer school leavers taking up professions in care. The use of NVQs may attract well motivated people who wish to undertake a particular training rather than obtain an academic education (Rowden 1992). The role of a care professional with NVQs should not, however, be blurred with other professional roles and, if embraced positively, NVQ training will enhance care delivery but will not replace the value of the professionally qualified care giver.

THE SPECIALIST IN THE CARE OF OLDER PEOPLE

The care of people with dementia will undoubtedly be a specialism of the future. It is important to have an understanding of what a specialism is and what is meant by specialist. However, Johnsson (1972) suggests that there might be one element that confers professional status: that is, to be a specialist the practitioner must have expert knowledge in the given occupation. In turn, an expert is a professional who no longer relies on analysis to connect understanding and take appropriate action (Benner 1984). The expert has a vast amount of experience and an intuitive grasp of situations.

Care for older people with dementia has many experts within the disciplines and this area of care can, arguably, be described as a highly specialised field of work. The problem is, however, proving that this is the case. Evaluating the work of professionals with older people cannot be undertaken using orthodox methods. Measurable outcomes, the use of technological equipment or discrete psychotherapy treatments are not necessarily appropriate, yet the skill of the expert in the care of the older person with dementia relies on the eclectic application of knowledge. The tools that the expert care professional has to use are the skills that are within themselves, which have been learned through many years of professional practice. The measured outcomes of the application of professional skill may be a reduction in or continued low incidence of aggressive outbursts without the use of physical or chemical restraints, or an improved score in a dementia care mapping audit. The key to unlock the speciality of working with older people with dementia is, however, confidence and articulation. Care professionals must be proud of the work they do and have the confidence and ability to present the multitude of skills they use in any one day to others and begin to consider creatively how to measure the outcome.

Working with people with dementia is an extremely rewarding and demanding speciality that will, one day, be recognised as being as challenging as paediatric medicine, acute psychiatry and child protection work.

ACTION FOR CHANGE

1. Take a look at a routine incident of care in your unit. Examine the incident closely and identify how many skills and observations were used to successfully carry it out.

2. Using the information in this chapter, draw up a quality plan for your service.

3. Work out how much money, in terms of salaries, is involved in a typical meeting in your service. Ask people at the end of a meeting if they think they have experienced 'value for money'.

4. Arrange, with a similar service in your locality, to swop duties with a member of staff for a day, every 6 months, and get them to critically appraise your service.

5. Encourage colleagues to use supervision sessions to draw up a list of their strengths and weaknesses with regard to skills. Use this material to decide on the training needs of the team in order to develop individuals.

6. Examine the last five complaints the service received, analyse the issues surrounding them and ask colleagues to brainstorm possible ways of avoiding future similar problems. From the list of possible actions, select and implement those that are achievable and practicable and that will lead to an improvement in the service.

7. Find ways to encourage the team to look at the service and their contribution in a positive light; consider putting aside time in every staff meeting for all members of staff to have an opportunity to tell colleagues about something they have achieved or an aspect of work that they feel they have accomplished well.

8 Ask colleagues about the reading they do associated with their work. Can all of them access appropriate professional journals and do they have time to read them?

REFERENCES

Barlow A (1990) *Transitions: A Self Assessment and Development Package for Managers in Social Services*. London: Local Government Training Board.

Belbin R M (1981) *Management Teams, Why They Succeed or Fail*. London: Heinemann.

Benner P (1984) *From Novice to Expert: Excellence and Power in Clinical Nursing Practice*. California: Addison–Wesley.

Bracken E and Davis J (1989) The implications of mentorship in nursing career development. *Senior Nurse* 9(5): 15–16.

Chapman A and Marshall M (eds) (1993) *Dementia: New Skills for Social Workers. Case Studies for Practice 5*. London: Jessica Kingsley.

Clark J (1992) *The Value of Nursing*. London: Royal College of Nursing.

Copp G (1988) The reality behind stress. *Nursing Times* 84(45): 50–53.

Darbyshire P (1993) In the hall of mirrors. *Nursing Times* 80(49): 26–29.

Dewe P (1989) Stressor frequency, tension, tiredness and coping. *Journal of Advanced Nursing* **14**: 308–20.

Donabedian A (1966) Evaluating the quality of medical care. *Milbank Memorial Fund Quarterly* **44**(2): 166–206.

Donabedian A (1980) *Exploration in Quality Assessment and Monitoring. Vol. 1. The Definition of Quality Approaches to its Assessment.* Ann Arbor, Michigan: Health Administration Press.

Douglas R, Ettridge D, Fearnhead D, Payne C, Pugh D and Sowter D (1988) *Helping People Work Together: A Guide to Participative Working Practices.* London: Macmillan.

Douglass L (1992) *The Effective Nurse. Leader and Manager.* Missouri: Mosby Yearbook.

Dyer W (1987) *Team Building and Issues and Alternatives.* Massachussetts: Addison-Wesley.

Ekstein R and Wallerstein R (1972) *The Teaching and Learning of Psychotherapy.* New York: International University Press.

Firth H, McIntee J and McKeown P (1986) Interpersonal support amongst nurses at work. *Journal of Advanced Nursing.* **11**: 273–82.

Goldstone L A, Ball J and Collier M (1984) *Criteria for Care.* Newcastle upon Tyne: Newcastle Poly Productions Ltd.

Goldstone L A, Ball J and Collier M (1987) *Quality Counts in Nursing. The Monitor Experience.* Newcastle upon Tyne: Newcastle Poly Productions Ltd.

Goldstone L A, Ball J and Collier M (1988) *Monitor, 2nd edn.* Newcastle upon Tyne: Newcastle Poly Productions Ltd.

Griffiths Sir R (1988) *Community Care: Agenda for Action.* London: HMSO.

Herbert R and Evans A (1991) Staff appraisal and development. *Senior Nurse* **11**(6): 9–11.

Hofman A, Roca W and Brayne C (1991) The prevalence of dementia in Europe: A collaborative study. *International Journal of Epidemiology* **20**: 730–45.

Johns C and Butcher K (1993) Learning through supervision: A case study of respite care. *Journal of Clinical Nursing* **2**: 89–93.

Johnsson T (1972) *Professions and Power.* London: Macmillan.

Kerrane T (1989) Staff Appraisal and Performance Review. In: Dodwell H and Lathlean J (eds). *Management and Professional Development for Nurses.* London: Harper & Row.

Kitson A (1989) *A Framework for Quality. A Patient-Centred Approach to Quality Assurance in Health Care Settings.* London: Royal College of Nursing.

Kitwood T and Bredin K (1991) *Person to Person. A Guide to the Care of Those With Failing Mental Powers.* Bradford: Gale Centre Publications.

Koch T (1992) A review of nursing quality assurance. *Journal of Advanced Nursing* **17**: 785–94.

Marker C (1987) The Marker Umbrella model of quality assurance; monitoring and evaluating professional practice. *Journal of Nursing Quality Assurance.* **1**(3): 52–63.

McSweeney P (1992) Does TQM have anything to offer nurse education? *Senior Nurse* **12**(5): 30–32.

Milne D, Walker L and Bamford S (1987) Professional coping. *Health Visitor* **60**(2): 49–50.

National Council for Voluntary Organisations (1991) *Changing the Balance: Power and People who Use Services.* London: National Council for Voluntary Organisations, Community Care Project.

Norman I and Redfern S (1993) The quality of nursing. *Nursing Times* **89**(27): 40–43.

Office of Population Censuses and Surveys (1991) *Preliminary Report for England and Wales*. London: HMSO.

Platt–Koch L (1986) Clinical supervision for psychiatric nurses. *Journal of Psychosocial Nursing* **26**(1): 7–15.

Rankin D (1989) Therapy supervision, the phenomena and the need. *Clinical Nurse Specialist* **3**(4).

Rowden R (1992) More input required. *Nursing Times* **88**(33): 27–28.

Royal College of Nursing (1992) *Skill Mix and Reprofiling: A Guide for RCN Members*. London: Royal College of Nursing.

Walton Sir J and McLachlan G (eds) (1986) *Partnership or Prejudice*. London: Nuffield Provincial Hospitals Trust.

Wilkin P (1988) Someone to watch over me. *Nursing Times* **84**(33): 33–35.

Williams C and Lowry M (1993) Professional development units. *Nursing Standard* **8**(11): 25–29.

Winn L (ed.) (1990) *Power to the People: The Key to Responsive Services in Health and Social Care*. London: King's Fund.

Wright S (1989) Defining the nursing development unit. *Nursing Standard* **4**(7): 29–31.

Index